# The Analyst's Desire

## PSYCHOANALYTIC HORIZONS

Psychoanalysis is unique in being at once a theory and a therapy, a method of critical thinking and a form of clinical practice. Now in its second century, this fusion of science and humanism derived from Freud has outlived all predictions of its demise. **Psychoanalytic Horizons** evokes the idea of a convergence between realms as well as the outer limits of a vision. Books in the series test disciplinary boundaries and will appeal to scholars and therapists who are passionate not only about the theory of literature, culture, media, and philosophy but also, above all, about the real life of ideas in the world.

### Series Editors
Esther Rashkin, Mari Ruti, and Peter L. Rudnytsky

### Advisory Board
Salman Akhtar, Doris Brothers, Aleksandar Dimitrijevic, Lewis Kirshner, Humphrey Morris, Hilary Neroni, Dany Nobus, Lois Oppenheim, Donna Orange, Peter Redman, Laura Salisbury, Alenka Zupančič

### Volumes in the Series
*Mourning Freud* by Madelon Sprengnether
*Does the Internet Have an Unconscious?: Slavoj Žižek and Digital Culture* by Clint Burnham
*In the Event of Laughter: Psychoanalysis, Literature and Comedy* by Alfie Bown
*On Dangerous Ground: Freud's Visual Cultures of the Unconscious* by Diane O'Donoghue
*For Want of Ambiguity: Order and Chaos in Art, Psychoanalysis, and Neuroscience* edited by Ludovica Lumer and Lois Oppenheim
*Life Itself Is an Art: The Life and Work of Erich Fromm* by Rainer Funk
*Born After: Reckoning with the German Past* by Angelika Bammer
*Critical Theory between Klein and Lacan: A Dialogue* by Amy Allen and Mari Ruti
*Transferences: The Aesthetics and Poetics of the Therapeutic Relationship* by Maren Scheurer
*At the Risk of Thinking: An Intellectual Biography of Julia Kristeva* by Alice Jardine, edited by Mari Ruti
*The Writing Cure* by Emma Lieber
*The Analyst's Desire: The Ethical Foundation of Clinical Practice* by Mitchell Wilson

# The Analyst's Desire

## The Ethical Foundation of Clinical Practice

Mitchell Wilson

BLOOMSBURY ACADEMIC
NEW YORK · LONDON · OXFORD · NEW DELHI · SYDNEY

BLOOMSBURY ACADEMIC
Bloomsbury Publishing Inc
1385 Broadway, New York, NY 10018, USA
50 Bedford Square, London, WC1B 3DP, UK
29 Earlsfort Terrace, Dublin 2, Ireland

BLOOMSBURY, BLOOMSBURY ACADEMIC and the Diana logo are trademarks of Bloomsbury Publishing Plc

First published in the United States of America 2020
This paperback edition published in 2021

Copyright © Mitchell Wilson, 2020

For legal purposes the Acknowledgments on p. xxiv constitute an extension of this copyright page.

Series design by Daniel Benneworth-Grey
Cover image shows a detail from *Diana and Cupid*, 1761, by Pompeo Batoni (1708–1787). Courtesy of the Metropolitan Museum of Art, New York

All rights reserved. No part of this publication may be reproduced or transmitted in any form or by any means, electronic or mechanical, including photocopying, recording, or any information storage or retrieval system, without prior permission in writing from the publishers.

Bloomsbury Publishing Inc does not have any control over, or responsibility for, any third-party websites referred to or in this book. All internet addresses given in this book were correct at the time of going to press. The author and publisher regret any inconvenience caused if addresses have changed or sites have ceased to exist, but can accept no responsibility for any such changes.

Library of Congress Cataloging-in-Publication Data
Names: Wilson, Mitchell (Mitchell David), author.
Title: The analyst's desire : the ethical foundation of clinical practice / Mitchell Wilson.
Description: New York : Bloomsbury Academic, 2020. | Series: Psychoanalytic horizons | Includes bibliographical references and index. | Summary: "A multi-faceted theoretical exploration of desire in psychoanalytic studies"– Provided by publisher.
Identifiers: LCCN 2020003316 | ISBN 9781501328046 (hardback) | ISBN 9781501328060 (pdf) | ISBN 9781501328053 (ebook)
Subjects: LCSH: Psychotherapist and patient. | Psychotherapists–Professional ethics. | Desire. | Psychoanalysis–Moral and ethical aspects.
Classification: LCC RC480.8 .W55 2020 | DDC 616.89/14–dc23
LC record available at https://lccn.loc.gov/2020003316

ISBN: HB: 978-1-5013-2804-6
PB: 978-1-5013-7271-1
ePDF: 978-1-5013-2806-0
eBook: 978-1-5013-2805-3

Series: Psychoanalytic Horizons

Typeset by Newgen KnowledgeWorks Pvt. Ltd., Chennai, India

To find out more about our authors and books visit www.bloomsbury.com and sign up for our newsletters.

*For Carolyn, Zach, and Katie*

*It nevertheless remains true that analysis is the experience which has restored to favor in the strongest possible way the productive function of desire as such. This is so evidently the case that one can, in short, say that the genesis of the moral dimension in Freud's theoretical elaboration is located nowhere else than in desire itself.*
—Jacques Lacan, *The Ethics of Psychoanalysis*

# Contents

Preface     xi
Acknowledgments     xxiv

1. The Voice Endures     1
2. If on a Winter's Night a Traveler: The Psychoanalyst as Innkeeper     15
3. On the Threat of Narcissistic Closure: Lacan's Mirror Stage, Cognitive Bias, and Narrative     31
4. The Analyst's Desire and the Analyst's Resistance     49
5. "Nothing Could Be Further from the Truth": Lack and the Analyst's Attitude     75
6. The Analyst as Listening-Accompanist: Desire in Bion and Lacan     95
7. Desire and Responsibility: The Ethics of Countertransference Experience     119
8. The Ethical Foundation of Analytic Action     155
9. The Proleptic Unconscious and the Exemplary Moment in Psychoanalysis     171
10. "And Let Me Go On": Desire and the Ending of Analysis     195

References     211
Index     223

# Preface

I was struck years ago, when I was a first-year candidate at the San Francisco Psychoanalytic Institute, with an idea that gradually I have come to believe has universal significance for any practicing psychoanalyst: the psychoanalyst inhabits her role as analyst with a specific desire that is all the more hidden from view when it is satisfied. In this case, I was in a seminar on adolescent development. The seminar leader was describing, with great enthusiasm, an interaction he had had with a teenaged patient. The details are not important, except that this patient, to the analyst's appreciable satisfaction, was coming alive in her work with him. After being for a time quite shut down, she was having her own thoughts and giving voice to them, and gradually she was risking having hope in her future. As Dr. S. was telling us this story, I thought to myself: "This guy loves doing analysis." And I could clearly see why. But his satisfaction and love went unnoticed, as if this particular analyst's desire in relation to his work with this particular patient warranted no accounting. A flower was finally blossoming in a well-tended garden, but the gardener's efforts and the desire that animated them were entirely taken for granted, buried in the amended soil. A strange state of affairs, especially for a profession that was established to explain the complexities of human desire and gradually developed a robust theory to account for them.

Perhaps it's of no particular moment that when things are going well in an analysis the analyst's desire remains sub rosa. While we might wish, from a rigorous, scholarly point of view, for a relatively complete description of the elements that make up a successful clinical process, it is often enough the case that when things are going well the wish and intention—the desire— that motivates the analyst's actions go without saying, and tend to be cloaked by codified technical principles and methods (e.g., analyzing resistances, interpreting primitive anxieties, mirroring an idealizing transference, punctuating signifiers, to name but some of the more common of these principles and methods).

On the other hand, the direct impact of the analyst's desire on the patient is of great clinical consequence when something is amiss in their relating and interacting. I believe that when the analyst is confronted by a clinical impasse of any variety—with confusion or boredom, or from a tense moment, to an enactment, to an ongoing stalemate—she is in a state of unacknowledged desire relative to her patient. That is, the analyst wants something she is not getting from that patient, at that moment, but does not know what this wanting amounts to or that she is in such a state to begin with. This kind of desire is registered as an unpleasure, a disquiet, a dissatisfaction. My use of the passive voice is deliberate because the unpleasure and dissatisfaction are experienced, often and in the main, as something happening "to" the analyst. This state of desire unacknowledged is usually tucked under the broad umbrella of the "countertransference," a state of mind in the analyst that is presumed to be caused by or intimately related to the patient's unconscious conflicts and struggles. Too often this presumption amounts to a well-worn and reassuring way for the analyst not to engage and come to terms with the desire that motivates her dissatisfaction to begin with. The nature of this wanting is, commonly, not mysterious and can be described as the analyst's wish that the patient responds to her in a particular way. This wanting is hidden from the analyst by any number of impediments that obscure it: either, as I said before, by a theory about countertransference, or perhaps by a theory of mind and psychopathology (that, one way or another, "the" unconscious has stuff in it that has to get out and go somewhere), or by an idea that has taken on special value through an identification with a mentor, supervisor, one's analyst, or one's analytic community. These moments of struggle and impasse are, to put things as directly as possible, more or less traumatic to the patient, and also the analyst. The less the analyst acknowledges her desire and takes it into meaningful account, the more traumatic these moments become for both parties.

The analyst's denial of the constitutive role of her desire sets up a cycle of bad faith in the Sartrean sense, as the analyst tends to attribute responsibility for the trouble to the patient; that is, the trouble is said to be because of the patient's "resistance," or "envy," or "narcissism," or "massive projective identification," and the like. The patient, in this case, becomes an object of the analyst's *ressentiment*, though such resentment is itself disowned as it is dressed up in the language of psychopathology.

That this state of affairs is ethical in nature is as obvious as it is profound. The question of the analyst's ethical responsibility for her desire (and the actions her desire motivates) runs as a clear and exigent through-line across the chapters of this book. This taking of responsibility is a necessary condition for any psychoanalytic process to have a betting chance to be helpful to a patient, because the analytic relationship rings emotionally false and is ultimately traumatic to the patient if the analyst eschews this taking of responsibility. As I describe in several detailed clinical vignettes, the analyst is often acting *prior to* predicated thought or anything we might describe as a plan of action. This we call enactment, in which the analyst "fades as subject." Owen Renik's work on analytic action and enactment, which I take up at several points along the way, has been of considerable influence in this regard and important to my thinking. Enactment is but one instance of the analyst's challenge: yet, *again* ... because it is an unending iterative process ... to take up that place of "unthought" action, what I call a place of absence, of forgetting. In Chapter 8, especially, "The Ethical Foundation of Analytic Action," I discuss these issues at length. There I make a clear distinction between ethics and morality—the former is resolutely first-person, singular, and non-normative; the latter, in contrast, indulges in a normative and universalizing impulse that has little relevance to questions regarding the analyst's actions and her responsibility for them. The analyst's activity is motivated by a particular kind of desire, but when this desire becomes reduced, as it often does, to a specific wish, trouble is brewing, the kind that can result in the *ressentiment* I just mentioned.

As I describe in Chapter 4, "The Analyst's Desire and the Analyst's Resistance," and further explore in Chapter 7, "Desire and Responsibility: The Ethics of Countertransference Experience," I encountered the challenges any psychoanalyst faces with regard to the practical effects of her desire on the patient and the analytic process through the influence of the neo-Kleinian school on our local community in San Francisco in the late 1990s and early 2000s. The effects of their influence on our group were large, to put it mildly, and amounted to a form of colonization; this history I highlight in Chapter 4. There I explain in detail—assisted by Lacan's concepts of the Imaginary register and the dual-relation—how my view on the constitutive role of the analyst's desire on the psychoanalytic process lays bare the basic structure of the clinical impasse. My differences with a clinical approach based on contemporary Kleinian ideas (most especially transference as a "total" situation, an expansive view of the countertransference, and projective identification as the psychic motor that makes everything "go") are practical in nature, because, as I explore in these chapters, without the category of desire as a unit of measure—as, that is, the key ingredient of the analyst's activity and impact—iatrogenic resistances (what I call the "dual-relation resistance") result, misrecognition reigns, trauma ensues. It is an historical accident of fate that I took this particular route into the question of the analyst's desire. There is no doubt that, were I part of a different analytic community and exposed to a different set of analytic ideas, I would have found another way forward into this nexus of desire, resistance, impasse, and ethics.

## What Is the Analyst's Desire?

By desire Freud meant the persistence of human wishing and wanting that not only colors our conscious experience, but also quietly (at times loudly) animates our engagement with the world and the people in it, and bends that world ineluctably in our direction (if not *under* our direction). Desire encompasses human experience that reaches far beyond Freud's concept of Eros because we can also be animated by wishes to hurt and destroy, and not only, as Eros implies, to bring disparate things together in a life-affirming way. Jamieson Webster (2011) captures this question of desire in more on-the-ground language: "Desire … is a movement that works in and through risk and failure … [and] bears an intrinsic relation with loss, with the delicate history of one's most intimate and frightening wishes" (21). Human desire is tragic in that it lives precisely where its object is not. This is how desire, always, goes on.

Human desire, fundamentally, emerges from lack, absence, separation—a founding negation. The simultaneous emergence of lack and desire I take to be an ontological fact about human being. This ontological fact has far-reaching practical consequences. Only in the wake of a fundamental incompleteness do thinking and speaking arise as distinctly human tools to mediate it. Only in the breach of separation from our important objects does desire emerge in the ongoingness of being a person, including, obviously, being a psychoanalyst. This ontological fact of human being is what Freud's exemplary story of his grandson's playing with his toy train and string—the Fort! Da!—is all about. His mother is gone; his toy train remains in her stead; play, voice, desire ensue. The Fort! Da! is the exemplary psychoanalytic moment in the structuration of the human subject in which signification, however semiotic and rudimentary, is cathected for the first time. I return to this fundamental scene and its rich implications at different junctures in this book.

One can only encircle desire. There are no definitive answers to the urgency it engenders. Regarding the analyst, her desire is hard won. It means, for starters, having been a patient in psychoanalysis oneself, in which, as Lacan put it most acutely, one undergoes "subjective destitution." Subjective destitution involves the analysand first in the struggle to free-associate, and eventually to come to terms with what is beyond the bounds of fantasy and meaning-making, as all meaning-making surrounds a hollow core or lack. In psychoanalysis we hope to come to terms, in some measure, with the trauma and contingency that mark one's singular life. This engagement is by turns beautiful and horrible, trying and sublime (in the classical sense of overwhelming). And there are desultory moments. We do this difficult work with a particular psychoanalyst, who, if she knows what she is doing (having been an analysand herself), stays with you through thick and thin. I gesture toward some of this contingency and trauma in Chapter 1, "The Voice Endures." There I offer an inevitably partial account of how these seemingly accidental moments—some directly traumatic; others in which people said things to me, each in her or his inimitable and often loving way—had lasting impact on me, and that together helped—there is no better word—me want to be a patient in psychoanalysis, and eventually to do this strange and precious kind of work myself. If all philosophy is unconscious autobiography (to paraphrase Nietzsche), and all writing is memoir—and this entire book is undoubtedly that—Chapter 1 is explicitly so.

The analyst's desire is a particular kind of desiring. It is not, for example, a desire to heal or cure. Nor is it a desire to teach or convince. Certainly it is not to judge, if by judge one means in the moral realm (i.e., right and wrong, duty and obligation). The analyst's desire abjures mastery: as a matter of principle, the analyst does not speak for the patient.[1] This desire is not under the yoke of a concept, a theory to be imposed or a treatment to be "practiced." And, as I describe at length in Chapter 3, "On the Threat of Narcissistic Closure: Lacan's Mirror Stage, Cognitive Bias, and Narrative," the analyst ought to be wary of overzealous efforts at understanding, and should be cautious about assessing a patient's struggles on the basis of her own. The ego is a narcissistic structure that tends to corral disparate experiences into false kinships and resemblances. This is a normal, endemic narcissism that we all live with; it is not anything to "get over" or "mature" out of. Cognitive bias, as laid bare by the psychologists Amos Tversky and Daniel Kahneman, is connected directly to ego functions that seem most rational. Bias is one way to understand what Lacan was getting at with the mirror stage concept. Narrative explanation, while perhaps an unavoidable aspect of psychoanalytic work, establishes its own conditions of satisfaction, its own tendencies toward closure, and will inevitably bias the analyst in one direction or another.

The analyst's desire is, ideally, for none of these things I've just mentioned. It is, instead, linked to a kind of embodied presence, a "staying awake," and a partaking of the free play of one's faculties to engage in an emotionally

---

[1] The analyst, at times, very well may speak for the patient, attribute mental content to the patient, or say something to the patient that she believes to be true about the patient or what is happening between them. But these are inherently partial (i.e., lacking) statements, and always the analyst is clear that these are her ideas; a failure of clarity in this regard risks trafficking in the confusing and contested world of what Lacan called the Imaginary register (see Chapter 3).

alive way with the person who comes to us to be heard and to be relieved from, or to shift into a different position in relation to, his suffering. These are general descriptors, important, certainly, but admittedly vague. To drill down a little further, the analyst's desire has both temporal and spatial features that in practice are indissoluble. From a temporal point of view, the analyst's desire is open and anticipatory, without an object in view, except on the empty horizon of the emergent, the next, the not-yet. I subsume all of this under the term *futural*. The analyst's futural orientation includes engaging with her own activity in the doing of psychoanalysis. The analyst is not only present, awake, and listening; she inhabits a passionate position and is willing to have an impact: she pokes, prods, and provokes, and she is poised *to be with* the unfolding consequences of these actions. The *at-one-ment* to which Bion directs our attention as a specifically psychoanalytic desire within the clinical hour has important relevance here. Also, Dianne Elise's (2019) work on the analyst's eroticism is an extended exploration of this passionate, desiring position, including the ways it is honed and enlivened by ethical constraints. From a more spatial, as opposed to temporal, aspect, the analyst's position is *gyroscopic*—dynamic, in a kind of tenuous balance, and always, even if imperceptibly, moving. A jazz drummer, for example, is continuously in motion as her head and torso are quietly centered over her spine and seat. A hitter in baseball is never entirely still as he is waiting for a pitch; he is always in subtle rhythmic movement as he waits. I write about this futural and gyroscopic position at length in several places in this book, most notably in Chapter 5, "'Nothing Could be Further from the Truth': Lack and the Analyst's Attitude"; Chapter 6, "The Analyst as Listening-Accompanist: Desire in Bion and Lacan"; and Chapter 9, "The Proleptic Unconscious and the Exemplary Moment in Psychoanalysis." Donnel Stern's seminal idea of "unformulated experience" is intimately related to these key features of the analyst's awake and mobile stance. Stern's (2018) searching phrase, "the infinity of the unsaid," captures the essence of the proleptic unconscious that I describe in Chapter 9.

From a relational perspective, the analyst is a curator of space. Like the innkeeper to whom I compare the psychoanalyst in Chapter 2, the analyst creates the conditions for her visitor to speak, to represent himself in whatever way he does. "Please, have a seat and tell me what brings you here." Everything in psychoanalysis follows from this inaugural question. The analyst's offer of psychoanalysis is meaningful only within this particular framing structure in which the patient is asked to give an account of himself—where he has been, why he has come, and who, as best he can make out, he thinks he is. These people are strangers to each other, and this strangerness becomes an indelible part of their growing intimacy. The patient's giving an account is highly complex and changeable over time, and is dependent on articulation—a "giving voice to"—within the analyst's domain. The analyst speaks as well, though her responsibilities are fundamentally orthogonal to the patient's. Importantly, as I stress in several places throughout, this giving voice to is much more a making, a *poesis*, a creating on the spot, than a revealing of extant mental content. Viviane Chetrit-Vatine's *The Ethical Seduction of the Analytic Situation* (2014), in which she explores the concept of matricial space and the analyst's ethical responsibility for the other, has been central to my thinking about these matters, and Chapter 2 especially could not have been written without the benefit of her extraordinary work.

## A Note on Lacan

I have been affected in an unerasable[2] way by Lacan's ideas, starting with an immersion in graduate school (see Chapter 1) and including his many-year investigation of what he explicitly called the "desire of the analyst." I tend to return in my own reading to Seminars VII (the *Ethics*) and XI (the *Four Fundamental Concepts*) the way I revisit, perhaps less often, *Moby-Dick* or *Paradise Lost* or *The Waves* (or, for that matter, the Grateful Dead's "Dark Star" from February 27, 1969). The riches found in those texts are never fully mined, a fact for which I am grateful. This book is, in important respects, a history of my ongoing conversation with basic Lacanian structural concepts: the Imaginary (Chapters 3, 4, and 7), the Symbolic (Chapter 2 on the speech-relation and other places throughout), the Real (Chapters 6, 8, and 10), and the intimate connection between desire and ethics (Chapters 7, 8, and 10 especially). Lacan's triadic picture[3] of human subjectivity and its relationship to psychoanalytic practice has been indispensable for how I orient myself both theoretically and clinically. His work is uniquely helpful in redressing the frequently encountered conflation of the layered dimensionality of the speech act with its semantic content. Lacan's emphasis on the materiality of the signifier and punctuation as part of an unfolding temporality shows that the speech relation within psychoanalysis is in no way reducible to "meaning."

But I find significant problems too, some of which I discuss in Chapter 5, where I worry about Lacan's emphasis on the analyst's position of absolute

---

[2] I am indebted to Rodrigo Barahona for this utterly right-on descriptor of Lacan's impact on many of us who have encountered and grappled with his *Écrits* and his seminars.

[3] To be more complete, Lacan's theory of the subject is quaternary, as the *phallus* (in the 1950s) and the *sinthome* (in the 1970s) are linchpin concepts that keep the three registers in some kind of dynamic relation.

difference, and Chapter 6 regarding Lacan's stress on the signifier's materiality which, though in many ways helpful, is in the end overly rigid. In Chapter 7, I home in on what I think is the central conceptual and therapeutic failing of the Lacanian position: that Lacan did not see the logic of his theory of the decentered, split subject (i.e., a subject constituted by lack and desire) all the way through to the analyst's activity. Worried about a "discourse of mastery," the analyst is constrained by concerns of imposing herself on the patient, that she should not mistake her lacking position with the "subject supposed to know" (imputed to her by the patient). Obviously, the possibility of imposition is an ever-present worry. But this worry is addressed, it seems to me, by fully taking account of the analyst's position as a lacking being, a subject of desire, just like anybody else. We are all symbolically castrated. The analyst ought never lose sight of the partial nature of anything she offers. All interpretations, to use Edward Glover's language, are inexact. The analyst is thereby *free* to speak. She is a curator of space, and can inhabit it generously, openly, because that space is structural—it is there to be tended, by both patient and analyst. This space gives rise to voice, to a "here I am."

The Lacanian perspective, in short, takes us a certain distance, but also limits our fuller appreciation of the futural and gyroscopic position in which the analyst functions most optimally.

Also, I do not discuss in any detail in this book, nor do I endorse it as anything close to a complete view, the harder-core definition that Lacan gives of the desire of the analyst. For Lacan, as I understand him, this desire is fundamentally a lure, because the analyst instantiates for the analysand within the transference the fanstasied and precious Thing, the *agalma* (so named in Seminar VIII), which in its essence is an empty object. From these ideas Lacan developed his theory of the *objet a* as cause of the analysand's desire to continue to visit the analyst and to continue to speak. The Maltese falcon comes to mind. For Lacan, in the end, there *ain't nothin' there*. The lack in the Other as instantiated in the analyst is recognized for what it is, and at that point the analysand is free to go.[4] As I write about in Chapter 5, "Lack and the Analyst's Attitude," the analyst is both present and lacking. None of this means that the analyst offers, in the end, "nothing," because in this nothing lives living, engagement, desire.

I have little doubt that serious Lacanians will have a hard time with how, in places, I have "watered-down" his ideas. I will simply say that when I hear

---

[4] I explore the arguably insoluble issue of whether a psychoanalysis ever truly ends in Chapter 10.

clinical work presented from a Lacanian point of view, I am repeatedly impressed with how "relational" the work seems to be—the analyst is open, encouraging, and supportive of the patient's efforts. It is not easy to square the theory of the *objet a* as it relates to the analyst's ideal position of "absolute difference" with the phenomenology of relationality and support that at least some versions of Lacanian practice seem to encourage. Like any good pragmatist, I take what I need and I leave the rest behind (to echo The Band's Robbie Robertson).

## Desire in the Contemporary Psychoanalytic Landscape

In light of the centrality of human desire in Freud's model of the mind, and the demonstrable ways in which desire—both patient's and analyst's—impacts every interstice of clinical work, it is surprising that much recent writing on psychoanalysis leaves desire at the doorstep of the consulting room.

Admittedly, one risks constructing straw men and women in any attempt at summarizing a psychoanalytic point of view, or in this case the contemporary psychoanalysis landscape as regards clinical work, prevailing ideas about the nature of the psychoanalytic process, and the like. And yet, I believe some statement not only can but should also be made about this contemporary picture so the reader can situate this book in relation to it. As I mentioned earlier, often we read in the psychoanalytic literature about a bundle of concepts that emphasize the analyst's inner emotional experience (her countertransference, broadly speaking) as a relatively unproblematic way for the analyst to apprehend the analysand's internal world and struggles. This direction in psychoanalysis (I was going to call it a trend, but in truth it is decades old) is not unlike that described by John Durham Peters, who in his exceptionally helpful book, *Speaking into the Air* (1999), chronicles the history of the *idea* of communication from the ancients to the present day. From Platonic dialogue as the "mutual salvation of souls" (45), to Augustine's incorporeal Angels, to Mesmer's "animal magnetism," humans have imagined, wishfully obviously, that a "psycho-physical" connection between souls is possible, though the various forms this connection might take have changed over the centuries. Peters writes: "The concept of communication as we know it originates from an application of physical processes such as magnetism, convection, and gravitation to occurrences between minds" (78). Whatever the specific connections imagined, the underlying desire in all cases is to bridge an ontologically irreducible gap between persons (or, for Augustine, between a person and God). This all-too-human desire is for a magical connection that fills a want-in-being, a lack that for some amounts to a profound wounding; for others it is the conditional founding of human possibility.

There is a fundamental reason why Freud asked his patients to speak. He knew that he could not speak for them, that in fact this was precisely the issue with which his patients struggled: that others spoke through them, for them, explaining away actions that from the young child's or teen's point of view were enigmatic and confusing, and often overwhelming and traumatic. This speaking for the patient was so total that their limbs and throats and vaginas spoke instead. Such was the nature of their suffering. There was no other way for Freud to gain purchase on his patients' anguish, and to begin to understand it, except within this speech-relation (of patient speaking and doctor listening); only in that way did the patient's suffering have a chance to change into something else. Each of us "speaks into the air" precisely because there exists an auditor—be it mother, sibling, teacher, friend, psychoanalyst—"out there," at some distance from where we are in space as we move air from our lungs past our larynx and into the air at any given moment in time. Human things get made through the ongoingness of such interaction between parties. Consider a newborn's cry and what gets made of it as the inaugural moment in his or her history of giving voice, because what gets made of it turns this cry *into* history, by which I mean the gathering memory of what we hope will be a tender recognition, and the developing trust in a loving responsiveness.

It is certainly true that Freud wrote about unconscious communication between patient and analyst and speculated about thought-transference (a kind of telepathic communication). His well-known conversations (and correspondence) with Ferenczi and Jung, and his "The Occult Significance of Dreams" (1933), attest to this interest. But these were minority reports within a broader theoretical and clinical effort that fully respected the individuated, embodied nature of human minds and human existence. However, regarding the contemporary psychoanalytic landscape, Freud's relatively sparse comments, while suggestive of something akin to what Peters describes (i.e., that some kind of psycho-physical process can definitively bridge the intersubjective ontological gap), have been taken by some to be the heart and soul of psychoanalytic work. In my reading of much recent psychoanalytic writing, I see a set of common tropes routinely repeated that seem motivated by such wishful presumptions. Here is one version of how this basic description goes (with said tropes in italics): the analysand is pictured as *primitive*, a person who struggles with *thinking*, or perhaps has a *psychotic* part of the personality. The analyst attends to her own internal reactions and feelings, namely her *countertransference*, which she *contains*, to understand the internal world of the patient, and especially the patient's problems with *representing* or thinking emotional experience (in another vernacular this is called the patient's "affect intolerance"). The analyst's countertransference includes her *reveries* and fantasies, which have special relevance to the patient's struggles, and the patient is averred to communicate these struggles to the analyst through unconscious, or *interpsychic* communication. Notably, because the patient labors to think, contain, and represent, the analyst is implicitly pictured as healthier than the patient, if not a therapeutic master; and yet, the implication of mastery (or at least the heroic) is unmistakable in some renderings of the analyst's activity. In the background of such a clinical picture is the implicit or explicit rendering of the analyst as *maternal* and fulfilling maternal *functions*. (There is almost always faulty mothering—a "bad" mother—to which the patient's primitivity is attributed.) While one can certainly find exceptions to this general description, I believe that in its broad outlines it is by now canonical, and is one that is redolent of the imaginary physical processes of which Peters writes.

The fundamental problem with this way of conceptualizing the psychoanalyst's position is that the analyst sets herself up as an ideal—a thinker, a processor of unwanted emotion, a metabolizer of the patient's "bad" parts. The analyst's inward focus is assumed to yield otherwise unobtainable information about the patient, who then is supposed to "take back" that which he didn't know he had to begin with. A related problem to which I dedicate a large part of Chapter 9, "The Proleptic Unconscious," is that of the reification of unconscious content there to be unearthed; this content, it is claimed, finds its way into the analyst's countertransference. This reification of content tends to solidify the imaginary (in the Lacanian sense) status of roles between analyst and patient (i.e., sick/healthy, etc.) that I just described.

I have always thought that this way of working and thinking entails a tremendous amount of unwarranted presumption on the analyst's part, not to mention substantial epistemological naivete. As if the analyst's desire plays no part in this "inner experience" of the analyst. As if the radical alterity that marks the difference between self and other can be bridged through looking inward as a first step, rather than looking outward into the world and across the room to the patient who has come to us for our help, and opening our ears to what he is saying and how he is saying it, with all that such saying may entail in the context of psychoanalytic work.[5] Only within this real time, on the ground interaction between parties, in which space is made to talk, negotiate, misunderstand, stammer and fall silent, clarify and correct, whisper and scream, love and hate, does meaningful and authentic psychoanalytic work take place.

What happens to the singularity of being of any given human subject if the analyst uses herself as the litmus paper, as it were, to "test" the emotional acidity of her patient's soul? How does this singularity—and the contingency and trauma that have marked it as singular—have a chance to emerge into the light of day under such circumstances?[6] I don't think it can.

## To Conclude This Beginning

When a person comes to visit a psychoanalyst, he comes at great emotional risk. He fears that he will not be recognized, and will remain, in some basic sense, a total stranger to the analyst. Such a person has learned through life that he cannot be himself and worries that the same set of conditions will hold true as he embarks on the journey of intensive therapeutic work. As the gifted and influential analyst Joseph Weiss might have put it, the patient has a desire to have his tenaciously held, unconscious pathogenic beliefs disconfirmed. He unconsciously hopes they are not true always and forever. In other words, the patient visits the analyst to come to life, to grow, if possible to flourish. But these "pathogenic" beliefs get in the way, and often take the practical form of the patient ceding his desire to the analyst in one way or another: "If only you would tell me what to do, how to think, what to feel, how to relate to other people, including you." Patients, in other words, tend to make themselves small in relation to the Other, in this case the analyst, by dumbing themselves down or in other ways complying, thereby implicitly idealizing the analyst; they inhibit their thoughts and opinions, get "sicker" through various forms of regression and somatization, and the like. They struggle to be themselves; they are searching for a space to be who they are, actually, and to give voice to this emergent experience of self, unfolding, in real time.

Will the analyst inhabit as best she can her lacking position and be, again as best she can, the curator of space? A space in which full expression is encouraged, validated, championed? Or will she locate herself in the superior

---

[5] Jacob Arlow (1995) called attention to this problem in his sharply reasoned paper, "Stilted Listening: Psychoanalysis as Discourse." I discuss the centrality of the speech-relation in psychoanalytic work in Chapter 2.
[6] Mari Ruti's (2012) work is of direct relevance here.

position of the one who knows? The position of the healthier one? The giver of knowledge in possession of a full presence? Will the analyst do what Freud clearly taught us not to do: speak for the patient, rather than assist the patient as best she can to speak for himself? Will, in the end, her desire as analyst remain hidden and unacknowledged, and therefore all the more traumatically impactful for that very reason?

Patients routinely worry that they are, one way or another, not "doing analysis right." The fact is that each person in analysis is doing analysis the way he, she, or they is/are doing it. Not some other way. Not according to a manual or script or how it's been written up in the literature. And certainly not according to the analyst. They are doing analysis their particular way, in their own singular idiom and style. In which their desire is made manifest, in as full an expressive array as is possible.

I sincerely hope that this book contributes, in its particular way, in its particular idiom, to this ongoing collective project that is psychoanalysis, to an exploration of its nature and its enduring ethical foundation.

# Acknowledgments

This book has been a long time coming, ever since (if I am clear-eyed about it) I stepped into Joel Fineman's New Critical Methods seminar at Berkeley in 1982. There I not only encountered Lacan—and the question of desire—for the first time, but was also exposed to a way of reading and critical thinking that, in nearly Lorenzian fashion, was "imprinted" upon me, and set my mind slightly awry forevermore. David Miller and Ralph Rader were also central to my early development as a scholar and, if indirectly, as a psychoanalyst.

By awry I mean in relation to my medical and psychiatric training, which itself had great value for me, and toward which, because of my Berkeley experience, I could not help but approach from an oblique angle. At UCSF, Mardi Horowitz and Bob Wallerstein were important mentors for me, supportive and encouraging of my scholarly efforts, and Bob's influence continued for the next thirty-plus years.

Psychoanalytic training exposed me to another set of smart and helpful teachers and supervisors, including Adrienne Applegarth, Danny Greenson, Lee Grossman, Maury Marcus, Owen Renik, and, especially, Joe Weiss. As a Robert Wood Johnson Clinical Scholar, my advisor was Hal Holman, a brilliant and daring mentor; he allowed me to find a project on the history of the DSM that continues to bear fruit in my thinking about the sociology of knowledge production and its relation to evolving conceptions of mental disorders.

I have been blessed with close friendships with colleagues whom I love and respect, and without whose conversation about psychoanalysis this book would not have emerged in its present form. To Arnie Richards I owe a debt of gratitude for publishing in *JAPA* my original paper on "The Analyst's Desire," and in supporting me and my work over the past two decades. Jonathan Dunn's wisdom, companionship, and down-home honesty have been invaluable to me over the years. I am especially grateful to Don Moss for his thoughtfulness and caring, as well as his willingness to tell me when (and why) my take on an issue is not especially well-conceived. Bonnie Litowitz has taught me, among other things, about the importance of editorial rigor, and has been of great support to me over the past decade. The Semi-Baked writing group (started by Bob and Judy Wallerstein) has been a rich and valuable source of encouragement, friendship, and feedback for many years now. The late Barbara Almond, Ric Almond, Terry Becker, Marilyn Caston, Joe Caston, Nancy Chodorow, Daphne de Marneffe, Dianne Elise,

# Acknowledgments

Sam Gerson, Peter Goldberg, Erik Hesse, Laura Klein, Mary Main, Henry Markman, Deborah Melman, Shelley Nathans, Rachel Peltz, Carolyn Wilson, Tzepora Peskin, and the late Harvey Peskin have all read and critiqued many of the ideas (and sentences) that appear in this book. I also want to acknowledge Miri Abramis, Martine Aniel, Michael Bader, Jan Baeuerlin, Lisa Buchberg, Judith Butler, Jim Dimon, Anne Erreich, Haydée Faimberg, Bruce Fink, Steve Goldberg, Laurie Goldsmith, Kevis Goodman, Jay Greenberg, Owen Hewitson, Israel Katz, Maureen Katz, Lew Kirshner, Jane Kite, Nate Kravis, Lucy LaFarge, Mike Levin, Georgine Marrott, Humphrey Morris, Dany Nobus, Steve Purcell, Steve Portuges, Steve Seligman, Donnel Stern, Tom Svolos, Abby Wolfson, and Lynne Zeavin for their willingness to engage in conversation and debate about psychoanalysis, including many of the issues that I take up, directly or indirectly, in this book.

From the beginning of this book project, Peter Rudnytsky has been a patient and stalwart friend, and a wonderfully acute manuscript editor. It was Peter's vision that led to the creation of the Psychoanalytic Horizons series of which this book is a part. To him I am eternally grateful.

Katie Wilson deserves thanks for her careful textual work regarding citations and bibliographic references.

Most importantly, my boundless gratitude goes to my wife and partner, Carolyn Wilson, whose support has been invaluable, and whose way in the world quietly performs excellence in whatever she does. She leads by example, and I have benefited greatly from her companionship for as long as I've known her.

It is one thing to acknowledge and thank dear friends and colleagues for their help in making this book possible. It is quite another to thank my patients, both former and those I see currently, for their willingness to speak to me as honestly as is possible for them to do. Psychoanalytic practice is an increasingly unusual one, in which the pursuit of personal truth is sought. I make every attempt in this book to honor those who have trusted me with their desire—their hopes and fears and losses, in the course of an analysis or psychotherapy.

Some of the chapters you are about to read have been previously published in altered form.

Taylor & Francis has granted permission to reproduce Chapters 1, 6, and 7.

Chapter 1 has been substantially rewritten. It was previously published as:
Wilson, M. (2018), "The Voice Endures," in *The Voice of the Analyst: Narratives on Developing a Psychoanalytic Identity*, ed. Linda Hillman and Therese Rosenblatt, Oxon, OX: Routledge, 50–61.

Chapter 6 was previously published as:
Wilson, M. (2018), "The Analyst as Listening-Accompanist: Desire in Bion and Lacan," *Psychoanalytic Quarterly*, 87: 237–64.

Chapter 7 was previously published as:
Wilson, M. (2013), "Desire and Responsibility: The Ethics of Countertransference Experience." *Psychoanalytic Quarterly*, 82: 435–76.

Sage Publishing has granted permission to reproduce Chapters 4, 5, and 8.

Chapter 4 has been substantially rewritten. It was previously published as:
Wilson, M. (2003), "The Analyst's Desire and the Problem of Narcissistic Resistances," *Journal of the American Psychoanalytic Association*, 51: 71–99.

Chapter 5 was previously published as:
Wilson, M. (2006), " 'Nothing Could Be Further from the Truth': The Role of Lack in the Analytic Process," *Journal of the American Psychoanalytic Association*, 54: 397–421.

Chapter 8 was previously published as:
Wilson, M. (2016), "The Ethical Foundation of Analytic Action," *Journal of the American Psychoanalytic Association*, 64: 1189–205.

# 1

# The Voice Endures

*I begin here, with an essay on the question of my desire to be a psychoanalyst.*

*What being, with only one voice, has sometimes two feet, sometimes three, sometimes four, and is weakest when it has the most?*

—Robert Graves, *The Greek Myths*

Dear Reader:

Let me be frank. I will say what comes to mind. The First Amendment, no less than the Fundamental Rule, underwrites my speaking my thoughts freely as they occur to me in consciousness. (It is of interest that I need the State to guarantee this right.) I'll do the best that I can.

But no. I will not do the best that I can. I will not say everything that comes to mind, all that occurs to me. The Second Amendment guarantees my right to bear arms—my right, that is, to my own defense, my right not to speak.

And so it goes with the psychoanalytic project: the hope to speak freely, my desire to bare all, comes up against the limits imposed by external structure and internal worry—the mechanisms, as Anna Freud long ago described, of defense.

"Let's talk" … so said the late Joan Rivers. Or perhaps it was: "Can we talk?"

Let's talk, then, about the external structure first: An earlier version of this chapter emerged from a request that I contribute to a volume on the psychoanalyst's development. It's something like an autobiographical project: Why did I decide to become a psychoanalyst? How did I develop my psychoanalytic "voice"? Who influenced me? What events and people in my life conspired to make me who I am and led me to be a psychoanalyst? Why do I continue to want to do this kind of work? What, in short, is my analytic desire?

These are not only good questions; they are the essential questions for any serious psychoanalyst to attempt to answer. The analyst's desire is about, fundamentally, one's desire to be an analyst, which means to work as one. As a general matter, we fail the profession—its future development and progress—if we fail to pose this question of the analyst's desire as clearly and straightforwardly as is possible. This failure is an ethical failure, because those who apply to be candidates at our centers and institutes have not, as a general matter, had this question posed to them. So hungry are we for candidates that little is required of them before they apply: not that they already have been in an analysis to know firsthand what the experience is like for them, and certainly not that they have begun to formulate for themselves the question of their desire to do this strange and increasingly rare work.

While the analyst's desire is an essential question to address, it is also an impossible question to answer truthfully, especially for a psychoanalyst. We psychoanalysts do know some things (while disclaiming knowledge of many other things). One of the things we know is that any kind of self-representation offered in a public forum (such as the book of which this chapter is a part), or in a private office (such as to a psychoanalyst), is an invested offer, neither pure fiction nor hard fact. Even if I am following the fundamental rule of psychoanalysis—that I should say whatever comes to mind no matter how trivial or embarrassing—inevitably, I choose to tell you some things and not others, all rendered in a particular way, in an ineluctable style. So what follows, here and in the rest of this book, is a complex rhetorical gesture meant, inevitably, to persuade or move you. At the same time, whatever effects I evoke are largely outside of my conscious control and are difficult for me to anticipate ... what you will think, or how you find yourself responding to what I have written. Whatever my manifest gesture amounts to or is constituted by, it is in some measure a faulty gesture, more implication than assertion of fact, more signifier and less signified.

The limits of self-knowledge are the beginning of ethics and responsibility, to paraphrase Judith Butler.

Let's talk, next, about the internal constraints. Which, upon even cursory reflection, relate intimately to the external conditions I just summarized. These internal worries have to do with what can be revealed—what to say from a personal point of view. And what it is possible to say from a personal point of view. I have a worry about what will happen with my words as they make their way to other people's eyes and ears. What about my analysands? Do I have a duty to protect them, in that I would wish their analyses to be relatively unencumbered by my "over-sharing"? What about my family? My wife? And what about me? I have, as I said before, a duty to protect myself ... from myself.

In short, we know as psychoanalysts, intimately and perhaps more than most, about this so-called freedom of speech—the seeming imperative of the fundamental rule of psychoanalysis: it is constrained by the frames (both external and internal) in which the subject is imagined to speak so freely.

Even so (i.e., in spite of all I have said in what you have just read), in the end I must take responsibility for how I articulate what I articulate. It's an ethical project, this effort at self-representation, this giving an account of oneself. And it's an ongoing project, a performative becoming, not simply (or perhaps not at all) a re-presentation of an already existing set of historical circumstances, beliefs, desires. Charles Altieri (1996), the literary scholar, says this: "For ultimately articulation is not simply a modification in language, it involves a modification in selves who have to interpret why they find satisfaction in it and who have to indicate what consequences might follow from that act of identification" (84). In other words, we assume ("that act of identification") that which we say and how we say it in a process of becoming ("modification of selves"), and in the process of moving into the future ("what consequences might follow"). There is satisfaction in this kind of self-making articulation. If psychoanalysis is worthwhile, it is worthwhile because of this project of articulation and emergence of self within the context and the constraint of the analytic relationship. And yet, in the end, as Judith Butler writes, "The 'I' cannot tell the story of its own emergence nor the conditions of its own possibility" (2005, 31). Within that "I cannot" the story is told and without it no story can be.

We speak of "voice." Not only the "who" of speaking, or the "what" of speaking, but also the sound of the speaking itself: the voice. To speak is to sound uniquely. The voice endures. Bodies change. Relationships evolve ... some continue ... others end. Fortunes are made and lost. Time ... waits for no one. But the voice ... its weird particularity, the unique way in which each of us pushes air past the thin reeds of the larynx, is the very signature of subjectivity. What I would give to hear how Laurence Sterne actually sounded! Or Milton. Or Melville.

The voice articulates. In the end, in spite of everything, as a person, or psychoanalyst, or analysand, one does the best one can.

---

It was 2005. I was at a high school reunion. The sun was setting on the Pacific Ocean as a large crowd of us caught up with old friends and vaguely familiar acquaintances in Santa Monica. There was a light, warm breeze off the water. At some point in the evening I noticed a very, very large man—morbidly obese—talking with an old pal of mine. His face did not ring any bells. When I approached the two of them I saw on the nametag of the very large man: John Cossette. I had not seen John in many years. And I could not believe what I saw: he was totally unrecognizable. His face had none of the features of the face I remembered. How could this possibly be? I said "Hi," and after handshakes and pleasantries, John started to talk. All the identifying features of his voice were instantly present—its lively cadence and mid-range timbre, his words playful and frisky, his sentences peppered by his high-pitched laugh. I was filled with that sense of pleasure one gets from the immediacy of recognition of something both familiar and wonderful, and I thought to myself: "Oh yes. This is the mark of a person. The voice."

John was completely transformed from the assured and brainy athlete I had played baseball with and against for a good decade in our youth. Now he was unrecognizable. But that spry and spirited voice—and his wry wit, his willingness to tell the off-color, politically incorrect joke—all of it was exactly the same.

Jacques Lacan spent his entire psychoanalytic career theorizing the signifier. If "in the beginning was the word," and if psychoanalysis is a "talking cure," the pivotal question must be, how does talking cure? This was Lacan's urgent preoccupation. He married the early Freud of the *Joke Book* and the *Interpretation of Dreams* with structural linguistics to create his version of psychoanalysis. Regarding the voice: it became, in Lacan's middle phase of theory-building, one of the five "object causes" of desire. The voice, along with the gaze, and the oral, anal, and genital zones, were remnants in the Real. These are ways the body lives on, and calls us, de-centers us, because it can't be completely domesticated by symbolic processes. So we find ourselves drawn to certain people who have a particular look or voice. We can't explain it; we are just so drawn (as I was to John's voice). The voice gives voice to the Symbolic but can never be totally subsumed by it. It endures in the Real.[1]

I think Lacan is right here, and these ideas are helpful clinically. But he missed something fundamental regarding the voice. It not only calls the other

---

[1] Lacan in the mid-1950s conceptualized the voice as hallucinated, a "positive index of the hidden truth of the subject" (Lagaay 2008, 54). Later, in his seminar, *Anxiety*, 1962–3, Lacan (2014) theorizes a more complex set of part-objects, such as the voice and the gaze—objects that the subject experiences from the outside, as other, but that Lacan insists are more absent than present. We might understand this idea by considering how alien—*unheimlich*—one's own voice sounds when listened to on a recording: "That's how I sound?! It can't be."

in ways the other can't control (this is the voice as *cause of desire* in the other). More importantly, the voice is the positive stamp of the indelibility of the subject, the speaker. To put it crudely: the voice doesn't gain huge amounts of weight. Nor does it become gradually more feeble or infirm. Moles don't grow on its skin, because it has no skin. Its organs don't fail, because it has no organs. In the end, of course, the very end, the voice stops, but not because of its own foundering. While entirely dependent on the body, the voice lives almost entirely independent of it.

I loved John Cossette. We met in the fifth grade at Brentwood Elementary School (only blocks from where, twenty-five years later, O. J. Simpson would murder Nicole Brown Simpson and Ronald Goldman). John and I played baseball against each other in Little League, Pony League, and High School. We both had professional baseball ambitions. But he came from a much more stable and successful family than I did. And he had a natural and easygoing confidence I both lacked and could only admire. His father was a well-known Hollywood producer who started the Grammy Awards. My father was an alcoholic who worked in the post-office in Westwood Village and delivered mail to the wealthy who lived nearby. John's parents were married, and had a big home in a ritzy part of Brentwood. (If John had lived in Westwood, my father would have delivered mail to the family.) My parents were divorced and my mother, younger brother, and I lived in a small two-bedroom ranch house near the San Diego Freeway. He came from French-Canadian stock and had an unassuming sophistication. (As an example: John appreciated early on the brilliance of the TV show *All in the Family*. I had never heard of the show until he told me about it.) I was a product of the co-mingling of two entirely different worlds: my mother's side was from Jewish middle-Europe and arrived in the United States permanently in 1938, and my father's side came to this country in the mid-eighteenth century from England and Scotland. One descended from the Bal-Shem Tov (so I was told), the other from Alexander Hamilton and James Wilson. You might think that such an origin would lead to something like sophistication; in me, it led mostly to a feeling of disquiet, insecurity, and doubt.

By the time I was five my mother had divorced my father. By the time I was nine I had decided, on my own, not to see my father anymore because he drank during visitation time and got into fights. He felt easily slighted by other men, and routine interactions could lead to violent conflict. At such moments anything lying around could be turned into a weapon. Coarse epithets tumbled unprovoked from his mouth, in a voice whose qualities now feel distant and inaccessible, but whose rage-filled content is easy to recall.

My father was an outlier of substantial proportions, so much so that I could establish, out of emotional necessity, a kind of psychic distance the lasting effects of which became clearer to me only in my twenties. But I also had a few things going my way that helped me effect this distance, a mapping that allowed me some sense of safety: I had an uncle and a grandfather who were both on my side and dedicated to me. I had a mother—beautiful, smart, and alone at twenty-three with two young boys. She was pretty tough in the face of adversity, and was committed to raising my younger brother and me. "Be thorough," she would say. "Stick to the details." This repeated over and over in her intense, insistent, take-no-prisoners way.

And I had baseball. I was exceptionally good at baseball. Better than John, who was pretty good himself.

I played organized baseball from the time I was eight years old until my junior year in college. I was especially serious about hitting. I collected broken bats from the teams (Semi-Pro, American Legion, and UCLA) that played baseball at Sawtelle Field near my house. (This was before the move to aluminum bats.) I'd practice my swing nearly every day in my back yard in front of the big living room sliding-glass door—every day for ten years. I read Ted Williams's *The Science of Hitting* and knew it backward and forward ("The hips lead the way!"). Williams was brash and cocky and wanted to be known as the best hitter who ever lived. In front of that big sliding-glass door I slowly but surely perfected my swing.

My first coach was Forrest Casterline, who went by "Cas." Cas was a middle-aged welder from Culver City. Totally working class. He was gruff, stern, and did not play favorites. He commanded great respect from both the kids and their parents.

Here are some of the things Cas would say:

"You should have had that ball in your hip pocket." (When a player botched an easy ground ball.)

"It only takes one. Hang in there." (When a batter, with less than two strikes, took a strike or swung through a pitch. This is counsel that is generalizable to many life situations.)

"Wait on the pitch. Let it come deep. Then be quick with the bat." (A crucial bit of advice that not only applies to hitting a baseball well.)

One time when I was twelve years old and the best hitter in the league, I had a game when I went hitless, the only game out of twenty I did not have at least one base hit. I was oh-for-three and hoping in my last at bat to get a hit, but it was not to be. Given that my home life was riven and sad, and my father was a bad actor and I continued not to see him in any official visitation way (he would show up unannounced at a neighbor's house and drink, and at my ball games sometimes and stand off to the side, away from the other parents), to be really good at something, in this case baseball, had by that time taken on great urgency. So when I grounded out weakly to second base to make it oh-for-four, I was upset. I veered off the baseline, not even trying to make it to first. I came back to the dugout, threw my helmet against the fence, and started to cry. Cas would have none of it. He said to me, in front of everyone: "Son, stop this nonsense right now. I will not have you acting like a baby on my team. You are twelve years old, not five. And if you continue on like this, I will sit you down for the rest of the game and have someone else take your place."

His voice: gritty and gravelly, authoritative and true. I said I was sorry, wiped the tears from my face, picked up my hat and glove and went back out onto the field.

It will not come as a surprise, perhaps, given the outsized importance baseball had for me in my growing up, that I stumbled badly on my high school team. Though I had considerable talent, I had more than considerable anxiety. This anxiety I denied, rationalized, made excuses for. I found myself consciously hoping for rainouts, or that the opposing team's bus would break down. Though I was a three-year varsity starter, and had some success, by my senior year I had played my way onto the bench.

Psychoanalysis is a peculiar practice in many respects. Perhaps the most peculiar aspect is the way an analyst goes about listening. We listen, roughly speaking, for the "other"—that which is unsaid, half-said, weirdly said, alluded to, implied by, inferred from, imagined about, metaphorized and similied, day-dreamed, improvised, stumbled upon. In other words, there is almost always an "in other words," a more to say, a more to imagine, to feel, and to speak to, again, furthering the analytic dialogue. In psychoanalysis, the straightforward, declarative sentence, while still important, has a minority status amid the myriad other voices spoken and heard.

But when it comes to a lived life outside the consulting room, and the voices whose uttered words meant or mean the most to us, we don't listen for the "other" in the discourse. We are hit directly, effectively, unequivocally (as in my moment of truth with Cas). We don't say: I remember the opaque manner in which my uncle gave me that crucial piece of advice when I was eighteen. He was so brilliantly allusive. Instead we say: When I was eighteen, after my first quarter at Berkeley, during Christmas break, my uncle Art, a child psychiatrist, casually asked me what I was planning on majoring in and doing after undergrad. I told him I was going to be a clinical psychologist. At this point Art became quite serious. He took me up to his study and spent the next forty-five minutes telling me why I should go to medical school. "You can do this," he said directly, after I voiced understandable doubt. "You can still be a psychotherapist, or a psychoanalyst. And you will have more flexibility in terms of job-choice, you'll have a more comfortable income, and you'll have more authority within the mental health field. Most importantly, you'll learn how to care for the sick, something that is precious and can't be learned in the same way in any other field."

This was the single most important conversation I had in my young life, because it was literally life-changing. I had great respect for Art Sorosky. He was a dedicated psychiatrist, always studying or working on a project. He was the first person to do research on, and write a book about, the sealed-record controversy in adoptions. The book was called *The Adoption Triangle* (1979). I can't say his voice was distinctive, but his words were, to me. I am sure if I heard Art's voice again I would recognize it immediately. But that won't ever happen: he died of a glioblastoma in 2001.

By the time I decided to take the necessary classes to apply to medical school, John and I had fallen out of touch. He went to USC and was not good enough to make the baseball team. I went to UC Berkeley and made the team as a "walk-on." I played only through my sophomore year. But around that time, during summer, I called John to see if he wanted to meet at Sawtelle Field where he and I had played together on a semi-pro team before high school, and against each other in high school.[2] There was a batting cage down the left-field line where, over the years, we had spent many hours throwing batting practice to each other. I suggested we get together for old-times' sake, take some cuts in the cage, and then go have lunch. I had a ragged collection of baseballs and several bats we could use. It was great to see him. He was his light-hearted self and in good baseball shape. We mixed fastballs with curves as we pitched to each other, took our cuts, and then went to the Apple Pan for lunch (a classic Los Angeles diner with great burgers and banana cream pie). As we said goodbye John gave me a book about Murphy's Law: Whatever can go wrong will go wrong. It was supposed to be a joke, a book of humor. I'm not sure I ever cracked the cover. The next time I saw John was at the reunion in 2005.

---

[2] For those paying close attention, the reunion of 2005 I attended was not my high school's, but that of our main rival. I knew many of those people from elementary school and junior high, including John, and wanted to see them again after so many years.

Medical school, it turned out, was not for me, or at least that was how it felt at times. The first two years were a hard and painful slog. I had depressing dreams of being wrapped in the same thick, translucent plastic in which the anatomy lab cadavers were wrapped as they lay stiffly in the Medical Sciences building at UCSF. I was a humanities and social sciences person (which is what I had said to my Uncle Art during that fateful conversation: "I can't do well in chemistry and physics. I haven't taken a science class since biology in the tenth grade."). This is how I thought of myself, and though I did well in my pre-med science courses, once at UCSF I felt out of place in a radical kind of way. The old anxieties and insecurities returned. Perhaps I had no business going straight from undergrad to medical school with no break, no journey, no risk. I don't know the answer to that question. After two years I petitioned the UCSF Dean to take a year off and go back to Berkeley to study English literature.

At this point in my life—age twenty-four—a number of voices claimed the main stage. I was in an important, if troubled, romantic relationship. My mother, thinking I had gone off the rails, expressed concern about my taking time away from medical school. Close friends were passionate about literature and writing. Confused but thirsty, I enrolled in a terminal master's program at Berkeley, in their renowned English department.

Imagine a cherubic, round-faced, short limbed, stubby-fingered professor of English with a sparkle in his eye and a gift for conveying what felt like the true significance, the "what is at stake," in a literary text. His voice was mischievous, playful, at times roguish, and always grounded in an ethical sensibility. When Ralph Rader was reciting verse or describing the role of Providence in the actions of the early novels, such as *Tom Jones*, he captivated the room. I remember his delivering the opening lines of Browning's "My Last Duchess," a dramatic monologue in which the speaker gradually reveals to his guest his having murdered the girl in the portrait they are admiring. Rader's performance, as he fully inhabited the weirdly detached voice of the narrator, was cold-blooded:

> That's my last duchess painted on the wall,
> Looking as if she were alive. I call that piece
> A wonder now: Fra Pandolf's hands
> Worked busily a day, and there she stands.
> Will't please you sit and look at her?
>
> (Browning 1842)

Rader was a neo-Aristotelian, which means he was very old-school as far as literary theory went at the time. While he read texts using basic concepts like "author," "intention," "action and plot," "character," "genre," and believed we all (at least implicitly) read texts with these categories in mind,[3] the rest of the department was being swept up by post-structuralist ideas, most notably deconstruction and Lacanian psychoanalysis. Michel Foucault (1977) famously wrote an essay titled: "What Is an Author?" (Answer: a sociocultural construction that puts a limit on what a text might mean and how it might otherwise "proliferate.") Roland Barthes (1977) developed the idea that a literary "work" is importantly different from a literary "text." (The former is a product—circumscribed, denotative, finished, complete. The latter is open and unfinished, connotative, a site of uncertain meanings that borrow and inform a network of texts, other sites of meaning.) These voices were of an entirely different order from that of Ralph Rader.

And reading Lacan was like going to the Oracle at Delphi: possessed of a burning question wanting a revelatory answer, one instead encountered the ceaseless mystery of ecstatic speech, a perpetual circling around an imagined object of desire, in this case something like "knowledge" or "truth." Ralph Rader (a mid-Westerner from Indiana) thought this stuff was nuts—needlessly hysterical and obscure, evasive, even sadistically provocative. But I was taken with Lacan's voice, the moments of hesitation and worry you can hear amid all the pronouncements and presumed authority. Lacan was, also, a first-rate reader of texts of all kinds and an equally trenchant critic of trends in psychoanalysis he thought were deeply problematic. These trends—American ego psychology, the reliance on affect as a primary signifier of meaning, the appeal of/to the maternal—left him, as he said many times, with a feeling of "abjection." Abjection—the state of being cast off, rejected, profoundly dispirited. A powerful affect indeed.

The psychoanalyst, while a listener for the "other," is also a practitioner of the Symbolic order. We are like Levi-Strauss's *bricoleur*: we analysts take what is available to us in the cultural surround, the symbolic tools ready-to-hand as we listen to our patients and make sense of how they are situated in relation to their important objects. As we listen we learn about the central signifiers and stories that they use to represent themselves to us, the way, as Altieri says, they give shape to themselves in the process of articulation. And as we learn more, we associate what we are hearing to images, metaphors, tales and myths, and artifacts of the culture in which the patient (and each of us) lives. "What you are saying reminds me of …" is not an uncommon way of offering a "furthering idea" to a patient, a building of something symbolically

---

[3] See Rader (1974) as an example.

meaningful brick by brick. But of crucial importance is that for all of us, including our patients, there must be places of disorder within this symbolic world, and it is these places in which the "other" can be found. My parents and their parents came from radically different worlds. My mother divorced my father when I was five. My father didn't fit, easily, anywhere. And within each of these moments of disorder can be found countless smaller moments (things said, actions taken, feelings felt and forgotten, fantasies imagined, desires dashed) in which the "other" might be found through a kind of "filling in," a kind of ordering of these shards and rents through the process of psychoanalysis.

D. W. Winnicott, of course, described this area of analytic work best with his seminal idea of transitional objects and transitional phenomena. Winnicott's is a picture of the very beginnings of culture as the child and parent transform the concrete object into an affectively significant one, the ownership of which is not a question that has relevance within such a space. That the psychoanalyst is a practitioner of the symbolic order is why the analyst ought to read widely, be curious about many things, and, most importantly, be curious about what he or she does not know. I remember well my Uncle Art's studying the lyrics of a rock album one of his patients had told him about. He wanted to know, in detail, what his patient had found so meaningful there.

I cherished my time back at Berkeley, and was transformed by that experience. Along with Ralph Rader, David Miller and Joel Fineman were major influences on the quality of my engagement with literary texts, and with psychoanalysis more generally. But ... I needed help of a more personal kind. I suffered from a bitter-sweet melancholy (more alluringly sweet, perhaps, than bitter). I had recurrent dreams about baseball. These dreams, which seemed to go on for days and plagued me throughout my twenties, were populated with the guys I'd played ball with, including John, and often staged in some way an impossibility: I can't find my cleats, or bat, or glove, as if I were reliving my high school nightmare over and over again. My father was back in the picture as well. He had been sober for a while, and would visit San Francisco occasionally. But he was just as insecure and ineffectual as ever. He was subtly competitive with me and unable to evince any sense of pride in my accomplishments. During my year back at Berkeley I started seeing a psychoanalyst, and once I returned to UCSF, I began an analysis, four times a week, which lasted seven years.

"Psychoanalysis is hard enough work as it is without making it any harder by your building up a large debt to me."

The words of my first analyst, a psychiatrist and a candidate at the time at the San Francisco Psychoanalytic Institute. This he said to me early on, when we were figuring out how to arrange meeting times and set a fee. I had suggested that I could owe him money, because I was in medical school and had none. His response so impressed me I never forgot it, especially the "hard enough work" part. I took it as a warning and a challenge.

This first experience in psychoanalysis was crucial in my emerging into something that resembled a person who was more than simply self-sufficient, judgmental, and flippant (all words friends of mine, in choice moments, had used to describe me). My analyst's voice, in spite of the declarative mode of his "hard work" comment, was at times halting, hesitant. He struggled with a stammer, and might get stuck on a word. Though he may have appeared wavering and wobbly, in fact he was rock solid when it counted. We'd fight too, at times. I hated it when he'd answer his phone during sessions, or ask me "How have you been?" upon my return from a vacation break. I thought he tended to interpret too generically: "You're afraid of intimacy," types of comments. I was not easy, as I struggled with an enduring sense of disappointment that often I masked with a pseudo-independent, cavalier exterior.

Complaints aside, my analyst said some things to me that seemed exactly right:

"You came into analysis as much to cure your father as to cure yourself." This he said to me after I had a dream in which my father was walking up the steps of the Medical Sciences Building, as if he were a medical student going to class.

Or: "You're afraid that [girlfriend's] natural enthusiasm and excitement will go off the rails, that she'll get crazy like your father did so many times, when he'd completely lose it."

And: "When I stammer you worry I'm not reliable, can't be trusted. That I'm going to fall apart, and you'll be responsible for it."

Someone who can speak to my fear of his falling apart is not going to fall apart.

My analyst was trained during a time when American psychoanalysts found a way to speak their minds in an unadorned idiom, with pith and intention, and without undue fear. Jacob Arlow used to say that we should speak with patients the same way we might talk with a taxi driver. Perhaps this might seem strange, because the people I have in mind—Adrienne Applegarth, Owen Renik, Joseph Weiss, among others—were "ego psychologists." And though the "one-person psychology" that most people associate with American psychoanalysis back in the 1970s and 1980s may have been problematic in some ways, the analysts I mention here were able to speak in direct fashion to their patients in a way that did not blame the patient or imply that the patient was up to something suspicious. I think of it as a kind of street talk. The interventions we typically read about now, or hear about in case conferences—a kind of formal, nearly arch way of speaking to a patient, as if proper sentence structure and diction relate directly to how a person's mind ought to "properly" function—were anathema to the analysts I am thinking of. They were not interested in protecting themselves, ruminating in the dense forest of their "countertransference"; they wanted to speak to the truth of what they saw in the patient as best they could, and go from there. Each of them inhabited a voice that can only be called their "self," or "who they are." They often used sarcasm or a joke; at other times metaphor, paradox, or confrontation. These analysts are among the lost voices of American psychoanalysis. Or perhaps, to make a larger point, American psychoanalysis has lost a particular way of speaking to patients.

Between 2005 and 2010 Facebook went from a small Cambridge, Massachusetts phenomenon to a global one. Over those five years, nearly all of the guys I had played baseball with and had all those dreams about managed to reconnect with each other on Facebook. John was among them, though his Facebook page was notably pictureless. The pleasure we all got from catching up and reminiscing about old times was felt, I am sure, by every one of us. In 2010 we decided to have a Pony League all-star reunion down in Los Angeles, where all the best players from that era would get together, play some softball, and have a party. And so we did.

John and I had had some phone conversations since 2005, and I knew by the 2010 gathering that he was seriously considering leaving his wife as he had fallen back in love with a woman he'd first met in high school. At the reunion he watched the ball game (such as it was) from the sidelines because he was simply too big to swing a bat or throw a ball. At the party afterward, he and I talked about some serious stuff (along with the usual cracking of risqué jokes): his brother's drug addiction and my father's untreated prostate cancer and recent death. The old connection was still there. Ever the Hollywood kid, he said to me: "When I saw you back in 2005 after thirty years it was straight out of *Field of Dreams*."

Early in the next year John left his wife. In April we spoke by phone. He had lost 50 pounds with a goal of losing another 100. He had accomplished this, he told me, with the help of a gastric stapling surgery he had undergone a month earlier. He was in an optimistic mood, feeling chipper, and his voice had that light and lilting quality I remembered when he was on top of the world years before. Two weeks later John was dead. I never heard the cause of death, but it was likely an embolism as he had complained about fairly severe right leg pain on the morning of his death. Pain he had probably ignored.

------------------------

Dear Reader:

I will leave it to you to cobble together, like a *bricoleur*, what I have offered here into something that might answer, if partially, the question of how a person such as I became a psychoanalyst. But anxious that I have not offered enough, I give one further story—another reunion story of sorts. It also serves as a parting story, from me to you. In this regard I am reminded of the Robert Hunter lyric: "The story-teller makes no choice / Soon you will not hear his voice. His job is to shed light / Not to master."

Around the time I was a senior in college I had been rummaging through my mother's files (unbeknownst to her). There I found an old letter my father had written to my mother's attorney in 1962, in the middle of their acrimonious divorce proceedings. The three-page letter, to my filial and literary ear, was quite a document. Here was my US Postal Service employee father, aping lawyerly language, rebutting every scurrilous accusation that had been leveled against him by my mother, via her attorney. Never mind that all the accusations were no doubt true. The letter was a masterly mixture of style, wit, sarcasm, and brash courage. I finally had something about my father I could point to and say: this is amazing. So I wrote *him* a letter, telling him what I had found and that I thought it showed not only chutzpah but also great promise. Maybe he could do something more with his life, be a writer, or a teacher perhaps? Upon receipt of my letter he called me, and the first thing he said was, "I always knew you'd come back to me."

# 2

# If on a Winter's Night a Traveler: The Psychoanalyst as Innkeeper

*In this chapter I describe the basic structure of the psychoanalytic engagement—the fundamentals of the work and the essential objects of the analyst's desire. Inspired by Calvino's title, I am inviting you, the reader, into my dwelling place for an extended sojourn, in this room, and the eight that follow.*

*The deepest Account, and the most fairly digested of any I have yet met with, is this, That Air being a heavy body, and therefore ... continually descending, must needs be more so, when loaden and press'd down by Words; which are also bodies of much Weight and Gravity, as it is manifested from those deep Impressions they make and leave upon us ... 'Tis certain then, that Voices that thus can wound / Is all Material; Body every sound.*

—Jonathan Swift, *A Tale of the Tub*

The psychoanalyst is a caretaker, a host, an innkeeper.[1] A stranger comes to visit, hoping for a respite, to take a load off, to rest his weary bones. This is not the fatigue of an exhausted traveler in need of a hot meal and a place to put his feet up. Instead, the wayfarer is burdened by a heavy heart or confused mind. Such a one would not be at the analyst's doorstep if not in need of relief from a suffering he does not understand. Sometimes such suffering is as intense as it is invisible, not only to outsiders but also to the stranger himself. More commonly, the stranger's journey to the threshold of the psychoanalyst's office is wayward and long, painful, frustrating, dispiriting. Relationships have been lost. Opportunities squandered. Regret has accrued

---

[1] Samuel Lipton, in his classic paper, "The Advantages of Freud's Technique as Shown in the Analysis of the Ratman" (1977), makes clear that from the early days of psychoanalysis the analyst has been, among other things, a host and caretaker of the patient.

as hope has dwindled. Perhaps there is bitterness and isolation, even moments of madness. Perhaps the stranger has had help along the way. Perhaps not. Maybe medicines have been used in an attempt to ease the stranger's pain. Whatever assistance may or may not have been offered or taken, here he is, hat in hand, at the analyst's doorstep. The story of his journey up to that moment of meeting will unfold, over time.

The person who greets the stranger at the door is not any old proprietor. The psychoanalyst herself is a peculiar kind of innkeeper, invested by the stranger with all manner of magical power and secret knowledge. This is a fact that, at times, simply slides past the analyst, as she prefers to see herself as the regular owner of a B & B. In this sense, among others, the analyst is a stranger to herself.

Considerably more is potentially at stake than creature comforts, though neither party, at this initial moment, can clearly see that future, let alone that a life will be considered in full. The question in this first hour is whether the two parties wish to meet once more. The analyst says: "I want to see you again." And the stranger makes a decision: he decides to continue to visit the analyst. At this moment, the stranger becomes a visitor. After more visits the analyst makes the offer of psychoanalysis: "I want to see you several times a week." The visitor agrees, and thereby becomes a patient. And the patient has a name. A name that the analyst will never forget.

The psychoanalyst is a gracious host, a listening caretaker. "Where are you from?" "How was your journey?" The patient speaks to her about his travels, his current concerns, his great fears, and his deepest wishes—in an idiom all his own, one that the analyst will come to know intimately. While the analyst is a gracious host—and part of that grace is knowing that she will inevitably reveal some of her own concerns and desires to her charge—her attention and concern are directed to the patient for his benefit. The vector of ethical responsibility goes in one direction. But benefit to the patient gradually takes on a weird complexity, because pain will be a necessary part of this meeting and talking, a key feature of this caretaking. Quite unlike a wayfarer sitting down to a hot meal by a warm fire, the visitor to a psychoanalyst's office will, at times, experience deep emotional discomfort and pain. Discomfort and pain that are, in the end, salubrious.

Though an innkeeper, a caretaker, the psychoanalyst traffics in strangeness. The patient visits. The analyst is there to be visited. A rate for each visit is agreed upon. The patient talks. The analyst listens. But the patient does not lie on a soft-linened bed and fall into a restful sleep. He lays on a "couch," looks straight ahead, and speaks "to" the analyst, who is behind him and essentially out of sight, about whatever is on his mind. Anything might be said. Dialogue is implicit, even if the analyst is silent in her response. There is the direct discourse of positive content: "This happened, and that happened. I feel this way and that way"—the normal currency of conversational relating between parties. There develops "the bond of safe company,"[2] the comfort born of the analyst's reliable kindness, willingness to speak truthfully, and to meet consistently. The patient sets up a home in the analyst's mind. An intimacy develops, but it is a strange intimacy, and that strangeness never abates. Whatever closeness comes to be, at the same time, something is inevitably missed, and this something is irreducible. In point of fact, this missing comes to be respected, maybe even cherished, as that thing which signifies the very humanity of the visitor, the analyst, and their relationship. What comes to be cherished most is the patient's singularity within the context of a singular relationship: that which he came to change, alter, get rid of, for whatever set of reasons. Through a psychoanalysis, there is a coming to terms ... a coming to terms with that which cannot be comfortably embraced in thought or cradled by words.

That moment in which the stranger first comes to the analyst's door and knocks will never, no matter what, be filed down through talk into something totally smooth. Running one's fingers over the planed surface of a life will always find a splinter, and not only one. The story ... or rather stories that are told will never entirely cohere. Even remotely. This is not only how it should be. This is how it is. There is one moment, then another, and then yet another. This incoherence is part of the very nature of the psychoanalytic engagement. The splinters felt and the stories told are held together by style and commitment—a dedicated way of being—not by narrative. This caretaking attention, this desire, from the analyst to the patient, is for the latter's well-being. The analyst's offer of analysis—an offer that is alive during every session, from the first to the last—places the analyst in a position of ethical responsibility for the other—the other that inheres in the patient's speech, in the patient as an other person, and for the otherness that inheres in the intersubjective relation and in the manifestations of the unconscious each participant brings to the analytic work.[3]

## Matricial Space

I want to be clear: when I speak of the psychoanalyst as an innkeeper, I am not speaking only metaphorically. I traced the scene of meeting, that a visitor

---

[2] I owe this apt phrase to my colleague, psychoanalyst Joe Caston.
[3] For a compelling and thoughtful exploration of the "foundational ethics" that the provision of psychoanalysis entails, see Humphrey Morris's "The Analyst's Offer" (2016). I discuss Morris's paper in Chapter 10.

comes to the analyst's office and the analyst invites him in. In what way does she greet the patient? Is the waiting room welcoming? Is the analyst's office at a comfortable temperature, or is it too warm or too cold? What colors are the walls painted? Are they adorned with art work, prints, photographs? Is the soundproofing airtight? How much natural light comes into the consulting room? And later: how is payment arranged? Cancellations? Texting between sessions? Emailing? These and countless other aspects of analytic practice involve questions of safety, care, concern, and while the patient has two clear commitments—to come to the agreed-upon sessions and to pay the analyst for them—as I said earlier, the vector of care and responsibility goes in one direction, from analyst to patient. Over the years I have had occasion to drive patients from my office to doctors' offices and emergency rooms. I have made phone calls on their behalf that they could not. I have had them bring their computers to the office to do work that had otherwise been languishing for months or longer. And I have been known to prepare a cup of tea or two.[4]

All of these aspects of practice fall under the umbrella of the *matricial*. *Matricial space* is the phrase that to me best captures the background conditions that facilitate—that hold, flexibly, steadily—the ongoing conversational engagement that is psychoanalysis. The concrete features of the analytic frame are at the same time signposts of the ways in which the patient lives in this particular psychoanalysis, and gradually takes up residence in the analyst's mind. At all times these concrete features are invested by the patient with transferential significance, though much of the time this investment is sub rosa, unarticulated, lived-in rather than talked-about.

The phrase matricial space, and the theorization of it, comes from Viviane Chetrit-Vatine. Her book, *The Ethical Seduction of the Analytic Situation* (2014), is an extended investigation into the strangeness and risk that inhere in any meaningful encounter with the other. The foundational encounter with the other is the mother/caretaker in relation to her/his/their child; the psychoanalytic encounter evokes and re-figures this original relational moment. Chetrit-Vatine leans heavily on Emmanuel Levinas's focus on the power of the face of the other, the baby, in relation to its caretaker. The mother, as Chetrit-Vatine likes to say, is interpellated into a practice of care for the other, her child. "The [child's] face calls me, interpellates me," she writes. "I answer; I am answerable for it. This response is made of this call that has been heard. Answering means being responsible, [being] capable of answering for it" (102). She especially emphasizes that within this relation

---

[4] For a brilliant and clinically wise consideration of these issues from a more practical—how to do it—point of view, see Ralph Greenson's "Beginnings: The Preliminary Contacts with the Patient" (2000, 1–42).

is a suffering that "cries out for justice" (33). "Thou shalt not kill are the first words of the face; it is an order," Chetrit-Vatine writes. "It is an order that comes from on high and concerns alterity, the menace presented by the very fact of encountering the other: this encounter connects me with the other in myself. It points me to the stranger in myself, to what is menacing, and so it disturbs me" (33–4).

Chetrit-Vatine traces this basic, foundational strangeness, potential danger, and fragility in one's relation to the other. Who among us has not, when holding a baby in your arms, had thoughts of harming the baby? Precisely because of this fact of human experience in relation to the helpless and harmless, Chetrit-Vatine invokes an ethical exigency to "do no harm" that simultaneously alerts us to the "menace" without and within that must be not only acknowledged but also respected. Love is not *something else* in relation to this menace; love involves the compassion and caring that live with it.

These conditions are all the more acutely present within the context of what Jean Laplanche (1999) calls the *primary anthropological situation* of infancy, that radically dependent relation between the *infans*, the helpless infant, and the adult caretaker. The psychoanalytic situation recapitulates the primary one, and so, like the primary caregivers of a small child, the analyst is in a position of ethical responsibility for the other, her patient.

Consider this meditation from Ralph Greenson (2000) on the basic fantasmatic configuration of the patient's encounter with the psychoanalyst. He gives imaginative content to the disturbing and enigmatic otherness of the other, in this case the analyst in relation to her patient:

> For the patient, the physicianly analyst is a powerful activator of the transference neurosis and the working alliance. The patient's image of the doctor stirs up memories, fantasies, and feelings from childhood of an authoritative, arbitrary, incomprehensible, and magical figure who possessed the power of the omnipotent, omniscient parents. It is the doctor who takes over when the parents are sick and afraid. It is the doctor who has the right to explore the naked body, and who has no fear or disgust of blood, mucus, vomit, urine, or feces. He is the rescuer from pain and panic, the establisher of order from chaos, provider of emergency functions performed by the mother in the first years of life. In addition, the physician inflicts pain, pierces the flesh, and intrudes into every opening in the body. He is reminiscent of the mother of bodily intimacy as well as the representative of the sadomasochistic fantasies involving both parents. (39)

We should not get too hung up on Greenson's emphasis on the "physicianly analyst" because he captures powerfully the mythos of the healer, and that the unconscious stakes for any patient choosing to involve him or herself in psychoanalytic work with a psychoanalyst are extremely high, filled with hope and fear, even a quiet terror, and entail great emotional risk.

Chetrit-Vatine situates the analyst's ethical responsibility within matricial space, a concept that suggests something more than a simple reduction of the analyst's position to the "maternal." She rightly wishes to expand our view of the analyst's ethical responsibility to a transferential field in which the patient's bid for the utmost intimacy, and the risks inherent therein, include but also extend far beyond the analyst's being open-minded and receptive, holding and containing (adjectival phrases that are routinely associated with maternal functioning). Crucially, within matricial responsibility the analyst is alert to degrees of destabilization in the patient from any number of sources, but usually from unwitting actions on the analyst's part that engender anxiety, alienation, or aggression—in which the strangeness of the other manifests.[5]

As I will describe in more detail in the concluding section of this chapter, the analyst's ethical responsibility for the "other," to that which is not-self, nonidentical, different, surprising, uncanny perhaps, includes an embrace of the analyst's fundamental strangeness to herself, and especially to the ways in which she unwittingly reveals her desire and its impact on the patient.

Within the matricial bond of safe company is the commerce of speech, a practice so thoroughly rooted in psychoanalytic experience that its structuring features can be easily overlooked. Psychoanalysis is a talking cure. It is structured on the *speech relation*—on the "Tell me: What brings you here?" This is the central question that shapes all others within a psychoanalytic treatment. The patient's speaking, or struggling to speak, is dialogically constituted, in that the analyst is an interlocutor for it. As the patient's interlocutor, the analyst "speaks between" the patient's words, and thus serves as a relay station of sorts: within the asymmetric, transferential valence that is matricial space, the analyst receives the patient's message and sends it back to him in altered form, giving it a new shape, and thereby offering new possibilities for meaning, thought, and commitment. In these moments the speech relation takes on an explicitly proleptic dimension, allowing the patient to cultivate "a transitional sense of self" (Goldberg 2012), less stuck, more alive, more open. And so, before venturing further into aspects of the

---

[5] Chetrit-Vatine is hardly the first psychoanalyst to demarcate this space of responsibility and repair. The entire Relational tradition, following Ferenczi, Sullivan, and Winnicott, among others, put this field on the map. But I believe that Chetrit-Vatine's work considerably deepens this tradition, sets it on firmer philosophical footing, and retains (rather than collapses) the basic asymmetry that structures the analytic relationship.

matricial which the analyst must directly mark, engage with and often speak to, I first want to describe in some detail this central activity to which the analyst attends.

## The Speech Relation in Psychoanalysis

If the patient is a visitor—which he most assuredly is—then he comes with a story, an account. This accounting unfolds multifariously, rather like Corporal Trim's famous "flourish with his stick," as indicated in Figure 2.1. In lines, and shapes, and shards, wayward and searching, told to a stranger who, over time, becomes a—and in some cases the—central character in the variously told stories that unfold. If the story told is really *stories* started and stopped, going hither and yon, then this speaking that the patient performs often exceeds what the patient intends. And this was Lacan's fundamental insight: that the "speaking subject" should not be confused with the "individual":

> Is speech like an emanation floating above [the subject], or does it develop? Does it, yes or no, by itself, impose a structure …? A structure that says that once there is a speaking subject there is no longer any question of simply reducing the question of the subject's relations, insofar as he speaks, to an other, but that there is always a third party, the Big Other, who is constitutive of the subject's position, insofar as

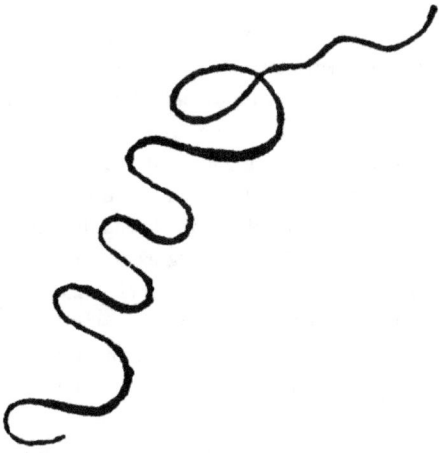

**Figure 2.1** Corporal Trim's flourish with his stick. (Sterne [1767] 1940, 604)

he speaks, which is also to say, insofar as you analyze him. ([1957–8] 2017, 163–4)

The subject speaks beyond the individual; the Symbolic exceeds Imaginary capture. This structural splitting is true for both analysand and analyst.[6] As an analyst, my effort, at a rock-bottom, fundamental level, is to create conditions within which the patient's talking has a chance to "cure," to be transformative, to change the shape of his or her life. I am not referring only to the obvious ways in which speech can dislocate the subject speaking, such as occurs in a slip of the tongue. What is much more common is that the act of articulation always, at least potentially, has a chance to alter, however slightly, the patient's subject position through the very act of articulation. In speaking to the analyst about how much he complains, the patient is already less of a "complainer." In talking about her need to "get everything right," the patient, by virtue of that very statement, is a little less in need of that very thing. These are subtle versions of Lacan's important distinction between the subject of the enunciation and the subject of the enunciated: the "I" that speaks is not the same as what the I speaks, and the "what" has a chance to change the "I."

Julia Kristeva, in her paper, "'Speech in Psychoanalysis': From Symbols to Flesh and Back," writes:

> Freud invented a "speech," a certain version of language which is perhaps not its truth, but one of its potentialities, and it is the formidable privilege of psychoanalysis to reveal it … And it is indeed this displacement of speech in relation to itself, this infinitesimal revolution, constitutive of our practice, which worries people. I fear that we are not sufficiently attentive to the exceptional singularity of "speech in psychoanalysis"— and, worse still, not sufficiently proud of it. ([2007] 2010, 431)

In this passage, Kristeva is alluding to the potentiality of a *felt difference*, an otherness, within the regular flow of speech, the infinite ways in which speech can be displaced in relation to itself. We might call this movement, following Laplanche, the ready potential of the enigma of the message—patient's or analyst's—through which something new might emerge. And Kristeva is right to call this displacement an "infinitesimal revolution," because in clinical work such displacements—such potentially transformative moments—are as numerous as they are, in the main, slight, at times modest, and often

---

[6] Regarding the analyst, I will especially take up this question of a structural split in Chapter 5.

seemingly insignificant. That they are constitutive of our practice—the very stuff of it—does, as Kristeva avers, worry people, by whom I assume she means psychoanalysts.[7] In most psychoanalytic traditions the speech relation is not only not taught, it is not conceptualized or theorized in any meaningful way. It doesn't seem to be "deep" enough, substantial enough, "emotional" enough. As if speaking were not inherently embodied. As if the very source of life—breath—is not sound's fountainhead. As if tone, pace, prosody—what J. L. Austin (1962) calls "perlocutionary force"—are not the heart and soul of any speech act. As if any uttered signifier has no independence from its conventional signified. As if, with a nod to Jonathan Swift, words lack "Weight and Gravity." No. We are all of us well aware that words can deeply wound and otherwise impress themselves into the flesh of the other. Yet somehow some analysts believe that the products of speech are merely the glossy surface around which or below which the analyst needs to go.[8]

Let's take a closer look at the speech relation in psychoanalysis. We will see that what may seem superficial—the diachronic flow of words and sentences—is conditioned by faults and slips in the structure of live speech that operate like trap doors, leading to other dimensions of deeply felt emotional experience. In these moments, an intimacy between the patient's speech and meaningful emotion comes to be; speech in these cases is anything but a gloss. Matricial space and the analyst's responsibility for the other support these efforts and are reinforced by them, implicitly, silently; through them the "bond of safe company" is made more resilient.

This "felt difference," this "otherness within the regular flow of speech," can be illustrated in any number of ways. The first clinical example I want to share is fairly dramatic—not, that is, slight or modest—in that a turning-of-a-sentence toward a different aspect, a different facet, had a noticeable effect on the patient and our work together. Early in his analysis, Paul was merciless in his criticism of me. "You idiot!," "I can't believe you just said that!," and other similarly harsh broadsides were not uncommon observations for him to make. I could never measure up to Paul's former analyst, whose technical rigor was both something the patient admired and that he felt I repeatedly failed to match. While on one level these interactions were unpleasant, they were not, for me, in any way disqualifying. First, they were *what was happening* in those moments. And second, I knew they reflected that Paul's engagement

---

[7] Though perhaps, as my colleague Peter Rudnytsky has suggested, Kristeva is referring to the "general public" (personal communication).
[8] This facile split of word and body partakes of a form of dualistic thinking—substance dualism—that has been roundly debunked in contemporary work in the philosophy of mind. Further, implicit in the point of view I am offering here is a critique of the routinely encountered and typically unchallenged binary of surface versus depth.

with me was serious and growing in importance. About six months into the analysis, Paul said to me: "I hang on your every word." I replied directly: "You hang me on my every word." He smiled and nodded his head. "Yes, that's very true," he said. Paul's smile was a clear indication that something new had happened. (This is the case more generally: unbidden expressions of humor and wit are often a sign that something new and important has occurred in the analysis.) And it was a key moment in this early phase of Paul's analysis.

One might reasonably say that I "named Paul's desire" (à la Lacan), or that I "showed him what he was doing" to me (à la Melanie Klein). Though basically correct, these statements miss the pivotal point: the felt difference between the two statements that was created within the reshaping of the patient's speech by my adding the word "me" and altering the place of emphasis within the syntax of the sentence. These moments, needless to say, are not, nor can they be, in any way premeditated. This is exactly the material that is constitutive of our practice: the real-time unfolding of speech and its infinite capacity to be reshaped, remolded. The same is true of moments of inchoate experience—so-called absence or blankness—that are sculpted, and thereby given inaugural shape and form, by words. The patient identifies with this shaping and reshaping, becomes intimate with it, sees it as his or her own, and commits to its truth. This truth is, of course, personal, and the patient's commitment to it is not of the conscious variety; it is more like an implicit avowal, a concluding affirmation, like a simple nod of the head that requires no further comment.

I emphasize this point about moments of felt difference within the speech relation because it is so easy, so "natural," to take this entire realm of analytic experience for granted and move quickly from it to two domains with which all analysts are familiar: (1) the generation of meanings, and (2) qualities of relatedness between analyst and patient. Here is one way such a move from the immediacy of the speech relation into the realms of meaning and relating might proceed: In telling me he hangs on my every word Paul is expressing a kind of anxious love for me, and through my adding to and altering his sentence, this anxious love gets flashed, or lit up, as the aggression I capture in my response reconfigures it. His aggressive criticalness is also reconfigured by that love and anxiety and so takes on different qualities and hues, as his criticalness is seen as a performative vehicle for his love. Relationally, Paul feels relieved that I showed I had survived his attacks, and did it in a way that reached him, and also in a way that he could admire.

Such a description of the generation of meanings and qualities of relating in this particular clinical exchange seems basically true, but it is important to notice that already I have moved to a higher and more general level of abstraction by utilizing and threading together words such as "love," "anxiety," "aggression," "survived," and "admired," none of which Paul or I used in that clinical moment.⁹ And none of which have any relevance to what transpired between us. It is true that this exchange takes the analytic relationship to a new, more intimate level; the bond of safe company *is* made more resilient. None of this happens without the analyst-as-interlocutor intervening at the level of the speech relation.

Hesitations within the analysand's speech are common. I often lay stress on such moments. If the patient cuts herself off in mid-sentence, I will ask her about it. Less commonly, a patient's hesitation divides a sentence in such a way that meaning is then divided as well: something other than the overt intention can be heard. A telling example is from Joan's analysis. Joan and I had been working together for many years. She initially came to me because she was often easily overwhelmed and anxious, and had recurrent somatic preoccupations. These struggles had changed for the better over the course of her analysis. Now, another summer break is upon us. On the last day before vacation she arrives like any other day, puts her purse on the chair and her coffee on the window sill. After lying down on the couch, she begins, "So I won't see you again ... until August 23rd." Joan's pausing after "again" is barely noticeable, and could easily have been unheard or, if heard, ignored. I repeat the sentence, but pause a little longer at the "again," before finishing with, "until August 23rd." "Yes," Joan says. "I heard that too. I may never see you again, full stop." What began as a prosaic accounting of schedules and dates suddenly and poignantly takes on a quite personal aspect. "Roland Barthes walks outside one morning and is hit by a bus," she muses. "Yes," I say. "And your mother ..." But I don't finish the thought as Joan interrupts me: "It's something that I still can't really think too long about, that she too is gone now." I don't know what she means by the second "too," and I don't ask. There is a long silence ... A siren screams in the distance. A dog barks down the block. Loss hangs in the air like a mist. Joan had been talking for some time about ending the analysis, or at least venturing into that territory. "We talk about my ending the analysis," she says finally. "I never really get anywhere with it. But now I'm thinking that part of wanting to end is to stave off the inevitable, that one of us has to go first, and maybe it will be you."

Analysis is rife with moments in which one word gradually generates a ramifying landscape of personal significance for the patient, and because this

---

⁹ This is also why psychoanalytic work is of a different kind from narrative construction, which is always an abstraction of that work. This topic is discussed in Chapter 3.

significance is known by and shared with the analyst, it becomes part of the specific analytic dictionary that marks and captures the history of the work as it is unfolding. These signifiers, what Bonnie Litowitz (2014) calls "stitch-words," are key elements that make up the growing symbolic field—a kind of domesticity—of this particular analysis. The particularity of psychoanalytic work can never be overstated (which is why abstractions and generalizations have no place in it). Only Joan, and no one else, ever said on that day and at that time: "I won't see you again ... until August 23rd." And only I, and no one else, repeated the sentence back to her with the pause ever so slightly extended. The same was true for Paul, of course, as he "hung (me) on my every word." And the same was true for Genevieve, a professional woman whose struggles with self-hatred and feelings of emptiness were matched only by her equally capacious intelligence and talent. Intense emotional pain—tunnels and darkness and death—was never far away. Genevieve is telling me about a student she is mentoring. She is especially impressed with, but also somewhat put off by, this student's "enthusiasm and positivity. She's so bouncy and so winsome." Genevieve then muses out loud about her younger self, reflecting on what her mentors said about her back in the day. "Were you in any way winsome?" I ask. "No, I wasn't. I was intense, and serious, and worked harder than anyone else. Winsome I was not." "Winsome" gradually took on a particular structural place in Genevieve's analysis: it was a signifier for that thing she felt she never was and could never be. At times it was that particular way she worried I wished she were.

Later in her analysis, when she felt a little more hopeful, and the bond of safe company allowed for a bridging of the occasional and inevitable bumps in the analytic road, Genevieve had found ways to, as she put it, "let things go," and "give myself a break." "I guess you win some and you lose some," she said to me with a wink in her voice. "Yes. No doubt," I said with a slight smile.

## Matricial Space and the Ethics of Care for the Other, Redux

These three clinical examples might suggest that the inherent play one finds in the psychoanalytic speech relation is simply generative of new formations, possibilities, and engagements. This is often the case, as analyst and patient are working in a felicitous, more or less positive interactive field, with matricial conditions operating in the background. This is what French analysts call working "within" the transference: through the analyst's capacity to maintain a *futural* attitude to what might emerge in the now-and-the-next, and not reduce the potential energy that inheres in the speech relation to things static (theories, explanations, abstractions), felt differences within the speech relation have a chance to come into being. This transference setting, as Laplanche emphasized, is, at least in the best of circumstances, *hollowed out*. In this hollow the patient is freer to fill the space with his or her subjectivity as represented in what is said, half-said, implied, or not said. Also, these clinical moments show that the transference that is positively conditioning the analytic work is not the same—and should not be confused with—the content of the patient's thoughts and associations. In other words, the analytic relationship can be quite generative as the patient is talking about something very troubling to her (a difficult relationship, let's say, or a painful memory). Not all content is an implicit comment on the analytic relationship. The analyst's caretaking function is in the background, operating in silence yet always present.

If speech's potential for other arrangements is, for me, a central focus of my analytic listening, it is equally true that often enough a different object of analytic desire must be addressed: this is the *patient-as-person*. In these instances, the analyst as caretaker, ethically responsible for the well-being of the other, comes to the foreground. Speech in these cases is *repurposed* toward naming and describing interactional moments that must be spoken to—given form and shape, as Donnel Stern has taught us—lest the patient feel further alienated and alone. Through this repurposing of speech the strange is then made more familiar. For example, we can easily imagine how each of the three clinical moments I just described could have gone south in a hurry; they could, in other words, each have been cause for an increase in the analysand's emotional pain and sense of alienation, disrupting the feeling of connection and forward movement of the analysis. The bond becomes frayed; the sense of safety threatened. For Paul, in another mood, at another moment, my saying that he "hangs me on my every word" pisses him off, because it sounds to him as if I am indulging in excessive cleverness. He feels even more put out, alienated from me, and longs more intensely for his previous analyst. Joan, let's imagine, is less open to the possibilities one might hear in her seemingly simple statement, "I won't see you again." In fact, she's more tired of the analysis than she has let on, until this moment in which I repeat her sentence back to her. It sounds to her, in fact, that it is I who is the more fearful one of loss. And Genevieve may have felt that my asking about her "winsomeness" was no more or less than an insensitive criticism of her, even a moment of humiliation, because I know her well, and that, more specifically, the self-hatred she can feel is precisely because she is not at all winsome.

One might say of these moments of disruption and emotional pain that the analyst clearly "missed the patient," failed to grasp empathically where the patient "was at," and misread the interpersonal context, the emotional tenor and tone of the field in which they found themselves at that moment. This description would not be wrong.[10] But my point here is rather that in moments of more or less traumatic disruption the object of analytic desire shifts from the speech relation to the patient-as-other-person. Matricial space is now in the foreground, in need of attention.[11]

These moments of disruption point to the *strangeness*—better, strangerness—that is always lurking within the analytic setting and analytic relationship. We tend to ignore or gloss over this kind of strangerness, what Freud in his early writings called the *Nebenmensch*, the "person nearby," or the neighbor-as-Thing. Who, "really," is this stranger who has come to visit? We tend to proceed as if everything is basically okay; things are moving along well enough; the bond of safe company is in fact safe. Typically, we disregard this experience or registration of some*thing* that is askew, that doesn't fit, that uncannily disturbs. (This can be true within the speech relation itself, as I have described in the previous section.) This thing *is* a Thing precisely because it resists domestication by narrative or thinking, though it does give rise to fantasy.

I mentioned that the session with Joan, under somewhat different circumstances, could have gone south in a hurry. I want to imagine how that might have unfolded, to bring out more palpably ways in which aspects of matricial space are, potentially, made present, when the strangeness and distress come to the foreground, and the analyst has an ethical responsibility somehow to engage and address these difficulties, which can at any given time feel extreme.[12] Specifically, the ethics of psychoanalysis involve the analyst in pursuing that which is elusive, beyond knowing, and must include the impactful effects of his own activity which can only be considered in retrospect, and partially at that.[13]

---

[10] I will specifically discuss the whole question of "missing the patient" and its implications for clinical work in detail in Chapter 5.

[11] Lacan was right to lay claim to the speech relation and its structuring effects as the central organizing endeavor of psychoanalysis. He was simply wrong, to be blunt about it, in so vigorously cautioning the analyst to refuse the personal engagement, and to view with great skepticism any attention paid to the qualities of the therapeutic relationship, reducing—in his terms—the subject to an ego. As I have already implied, such attention may well be necessary, especially when disruptions (for whatever reason) and their effects must be recognized and talked about.

[12] This case is "imagined" for purposes of confidentiality. It is similar in form to actual analyses in my practice. The content is changed, but the dynamic structure of the interaction is close to the same as what "actually happened."

[13] This issue is the subject of Chapter 8, "The Ethical Foundation of Analytic Action."

Let's say my emphasizing the brief pause after "I won't see you again ..." more than annoys Joan. She is clearly upset. The clinical interaction has, in fact, grown much more difficult, and the suddenness with which the emotional tenor changed is part of the strangeness, the risk, even the potential "menace" alive in the background of any psychoanalytic interaction.

"You haven't helped me," Joan says, "to really talk about how you and I can end this analysis. Instead, when you get the chance, like today, you emphasize how this is my struggle, not our struggle or, maybe more to the point, your struggle."

Surprised that this is where we now find ourselves, I am quiet for a bit, sensing that something grave and serious is unfolding. Finally, I say: "Maybe you're right, about my struggle I mean. Obviously, what I said upset you ... What else do you notice, or have you noticed, about how I might be struggling with our ending?"

"I don't know ... I don't feel like talking about it ... It's something about the way that, lately, you've greeted me in the waiting room, when you come to get me. You're a little more reserved, held back, kind of flat."

"Oh." I am, again, surprised to hear this, and consider whether she might be right. Here my decentered position as analyst is clear: Could I possibly know how, in fact, and in what way I have greeted Joan lately? I try as best I can to be with this absent place, this "how could I possibly know?," follow her lead, and see where it goes.

"Yes. I hadn't really thought about it before now as something that might mean something. I don't like it." Joan is getting more upset, and tearful.

The room seems wobbly. The light uncertain. The bond of safe company clearly shaken. "Now that we're here, and you're letting me know about it, the waiting room greeting I mean, what do you make of it?"

"That you are having a hard time saying goodbye to me, just like I'm having a hard time really considering stopping my analysis."

"Saying goodbye to me."

"Yes. And, also, that you're having the office painted during this break." I had told Joan, and the rest of my patients, that new carpet would be installed and the walls painted during the vacation break.

I now get how these features of the matricial setting are suddenly front and center: the waiting room, my greeting, my office changing through new paint and carpet. I say: "Uh-hmm ... As if I've already said goodbye to you inside without doing any of the real work of actually saying goodbye and helping you do that work too. Instead, I'm painting my office as if I'm readying it for a new analytic patient."

"Right. That's what it feels like to me, and that's what I worry about. It's tremendously upsetting. I just want to say, 'Fuck you, okay? We're done. Maybe this should be our last session.'" Joan cries more.

Though I don't, at this point in the hour, think Joan means what she just said about this being our last session, the constructed nature of psychoanalytic work—that it is based, as it were, on a handshake—and the fact that she voluntarily comes to visit me, and, further, that bad feelings have so easily overtaken both of us ... all of this together creates the distinct and unmistakable feeling that our entire effort, all the years of analytic work, could fall apart in an instant. The ground simply swallows us up and we're gone. This kind of experience is at the heart of the strangeness of any human interaction, including psychoanalysis.

It is also why psychoanalysis is, often, demanding work. It takes effort of both heart and mind to be with moments like this, and attend as best one can to what is happening in the now-and-the-next of the unfolding hour. In this session with Joan, what is usually in the background, taken for granted, is very present before us. My ethical responsibility for the other, for her care, means that I am also responsible for my actions, including especially those whose significance and meaning have eluded me. With Joan, the imminent summer break, my waiting room greeting, and my office being painted together created the complex emotional field that we didn't know we were walking in, all conditioned by the now looming question of ending the analysis. When she takes note of my waiting-room greeting, I then take note of it too. The same with my office being painted during the vacation break. These are actions I am doing, the impact of which I am responsible for. The proximate cause of her upset was my laying stress on her words and the gaps in-between them within the larger context I have related. It may appear that we are far away from anything to do with the speech relation as I described it earlier in this chapter. But this is only superficially true. In fact, speech has been repurposed, put into service as a way to mark these difficult moments between Joan and me with a tone of honesty, open-mindedness, and tenderness.

I extended this clinical vignette of Joan to give the reader a palpable sense of how I reoriented my analytic desire to attend to her—and my—distress as a way of explicating the matricial space and the analyst's ethical responsibility for the other. As I have attempted to demonstrate in this chapter, matricial space and the ethics of care for the other are, in fact, never-not-present as the field condition of any psychoanalytic treatment.

But the lure of identity—how we like to think about ourselves, our "ego-cathexes," the stories we tell about ourselves and our patients—is ever-present. We wish to abjure the strangeness in ourselves and in the analytic relationship. As Laplanche said: All analysts struggle with "the constant threat of narcissistic closure" (1999, 81). This is where we will next turn, to the question of narcissism and the ego, bias, and what Lacan was getting at with the Mirror Stage.

# 3

# On the Threat of Narcissistic Closure: Lacan's Mirror Stage, Cognitive Bias, and Narrative

*In Chapter 2 I described in detail the two realms of psychoanalytic experience that I focus on as an analyst: the speech relation, and the conditioning background to that work, namely matricial space and the ethics of care for the other that the matricial requires. As will become gradually clearer in subsequent chapters, the analyst's desire is not reducible to specific objects of attention. Such a reduction risks immobilizing, at least relatively speaking, a spirited, alive kind of working in which the analyst's desire is tracking what is happening in the "rolling forward of the now," what I term the futural. In Chapter 6, especially, where I consider the status of desire in Bion and Lacan, this analytic position, which is in fact an ideal one—aspirational, asymptotic—the reader will get a better sense of the radical openness of the analyst's desire. In this chapter I focus on desire's antagonist, namely the ego and its fundamentally narcissistic nature.*

While it is difficult to nail down descriptively what the analyst's desire is, we can say right away what it is not. It is not based on any illusory and evanescent inventions that are marked by what Lacan called the Imaginary order, the realm, that is, of narcissism and the ego. Narrative explanation is one such invention. To the extent that the story told is stable, coherent, and invested with value, it risks being not only a salve for the analyst's uncertainty and the strangeness of the analytic encounter. An overly enthusiastic narrative approach to analytic work—in which the analyst may believe he is working solely in the Symbolic register—can also take on Imaginary features if the analyst invests the gathering story with a privileged explanatory power. As I will describe later in this chapter, robust narratives create their own conditions of satisfaction as they tend to constrain what is allowed to be possible, whether by being simply thinkable or experienced in some other way.

More basically, the ego's illusory and evanescent inventions involve various forms of idealization, both necessary and false, that are at once captivating and reassuring. These inventions establish a set of more or less inescapable—perhaps at times impassable—conditions for a person who imagines being a psychoanalyst. Idealization often takes the form of self-images that an analyst may have regarding his "analytic identity," an identity conferred upon him by the psychoanalytic institute or association. Recently, while I was cleaning out my office closet, I found my membership certificate from the American Psychoanalytic Association. Still in the folder in which I received it back in 1997, it was pristine (no coffee stains) and looked quite official. I felt some pride, for sure, even if, at the same time, I was aware that the American Psychoanalytic Association was/is a troubled entity, with a declining and aging membership, and plagued by seemingly never-ending intramural tensions. And even if the American (as it is known) were an enduringly venerable and robust association, this fact would not matter regarding my analytic desire, though the pride I felt at finding my certificate might then have been greater than in fact it was.

There are, of course, more immediately personal ways in which a psychoanalytic identity comes into being, usually through special relationships with one's analyst, or a supervisor, or an analytic figure that enthralls because of his or her capacity for demonstrations of clinical brilliance in supervision or a public setting. In truth, like visions in the night, such attachments often come and go. Learning from other analysts is, obviously, of crucial importance for any clinician. I am speaking here of idealization, a phenomenon to which few analysts are immune. It doesn't seem to matter that today's compelling psychoanalytic "master" is entirely incompatible, from a clinical or theoretical point of view, from last year's well-feted analytic celebrity. Our desire to identify—to admire and idealize—is that great, and can be that fickle.

Or, consider the phrase "analytic conviction." The analyst is supposed to have it. To have it is to have confidence, as a general matter, that psychoanalysis works, is helpful, and, most importantly, is the treatment that is indicated for the person sitting before us in our consulting room. Conviction suggests that our place as a psychoanalyst is secure, our seat warm, our vision clear. One sees courses in psychoanalytic institutes on "Building a Psychoanalytic Identity," on "Psychoanalytic Conviction," and about "Conversion to Psychoanalysis from Psychotherapy." The word "conversion" might stir feelings of concern, as the religious connotations are hard to miss.

A particularly powerful way to summarize what I have just briefly described is that all analysts, as Laplanche (1999) has said, work "under the constant threat of narcissistic closure" (81). This basic threat cannot be too strongly stated, nor can it be too easily assented to lest we not give this threat its due, which is substantial. Notice that even if I have my eye on the lures that identity and idealization seem to offer, and even if have developed a hard-earned warning system regarding their dangers, this position itself can ossify into something overvalued and fixed. This is perhaps why Laplanche emphasizes the "constant threat" of these illusory and evanescent constructions. Any position the analyst maintains, especially one based on psychoanalytic theory that one avers to the true—really believes in, and really thinks is right in the veridical sense of the word—can fall prey to excessive narcissistic investment, and serve the purposes of shoring up the analyst's wavering ego. The analyst's desire is always a position contrary to her narcissism in whatever form that investment takes.

I will spend the next few pages describing this "threat of narcissistic closure," and so will consider in detail Lacan's theory of the mirror stage and the narcissistic basis of the ego. Mirroring, from this point of view, is necessarily a closing up, a binding, and the ego's efforts in this regard link up in surprising ways with the extraordinarily influential work on cognitive bias by Amos Tversky and Daniel Kahneman. Psychoanalysts should know about this work. I'll spend some time explaining it, and its relevance to psychoanalysts. Finally, I consider the question of narrative in light of what has come before.

"The threat of narcissistic closure." Laplanche's use of the word "threat" may seem, perhaps, an unfortunate choice, because it implies that we analysts require a certain vigilance with respect to some bad thing looming from the "outside." Laplanche did not at all intend this implication; he understood as well as anyone that each of us lives with a natural narcissism, a self-preservative and self-supporting effort that stretches from our seeking nutritional sustenance to our exercising the cognitive capacities of memory and judgment. For the psychoanalyst, however, this aspect of subjective experience, in which my personhood can feel to be at stake, in which "who I am" is an issue ... yes, this aspect can present the analyst with significant problems. I emphasize the tentative "can present," because this state of affairs is substantially dependent on the analyst's state of mind at the moment and whether her desire is mobile ... open ... or, if, by being reduced to a specific wish, is fixed or closed. In the former case, the open mobility of the analyst's desire is always, potentially, in proximity to manifestations of the unconscious in which a significant difference—something other or surprising or strange or witty—is realized in the now-and-the-next.[1] In the

[1] When Laplanche writes of the enigma of the message, a kind of otherness, he emphasizes its foreignness, its strangeness.

latter case of a fixed analytic field, the analyst is caught, or caught up, in worries about identity, role, and self-image precisely in relation to the other *person*, in this case, the analysand, but also, not uncommonly, in relation to the ambivalently admired "master" whose work the analyst feels compelled to imitate.

In fact, the perpetual instability of identity and of the identifications on which identity is built arises precisely because *identity* and *the other*—captured in the seemingly tautological statements, "who I am," or, "I am who"—sit in a perpetually uneasy relation. This is Lacan's core insight about the nature of the ego: the ego arises and is maintained in a mirroring, wavering, and rivalrous relation with the other ... an "other" that is a mobile, fungible element of the self. In this light, Laplanche's use of the word "threat" aptly captures this feature of identity, one that marks its very constitution. Narcissus's looking at his glassy visage in a pool of water is, as we know, a closed system—static, airless, more dead than alive, all of which belies the ecstasy he feels at that moment he is with himself.

## What Lacan Was Getting at with the Mirror Stage

The source of Laplanche's warning about narcissism and the analyst,[2] as many readers know, is Lacan's theory of the mirror stage as the founding story of the ego's fate, based on its irreducibly narcissistic nature. In Lacan's mirror stage we find a density of theoretical insight—a condensation in the Freudian sense—that itself is an interpretation of Freud's theory of the ego. In "On Narcissism" (1914), Freud posits a dual instinct theory in which the ego (i.e., self-preservative) instincts are in perpetual tension with the sexual instincts. Self-preservation and sexual desire are in conflict.

Later, in *The Ego and the Id* (1923), Freud asserts:

> The ego is first and foremost a bodily ego; it is not merely a surface entity, but is itself the projection of a surface. If we wish to find an anatomical analogy for it we can best identify it with the "cortical homunculus" of the anatomists, which stands on its head in the cortex, sticks up its heels,

---

[2] In fact, in Laplanche's paper, "The Unfinished Copernican Revolution" (1999), he is making a point about Freud's theory-building that extends far beyond the clinical: that Freud's fundamental emphasis on the decentered subject in relation to the unconscious "closes in on itself" in a recentering "Ptolemaic" move, and, therefore, continually abjures its revolutionary insights. "Narcissism," Laplanche writes, "remains key to the problem" (82).

faces backwards and, as we know, has its speech-area on the left-hand side. (31)

Regarding the features of one's character, Freud speaks to the importance of identification, a way the young person takes on the qualities of important others with whom he is involved: "The character of the ego is a precipitate of abandoned object-cathexes and it contains the history of those object-choices" (29).[3]

From these basic Freudian claims (leavened with some Hegel and Konrad Lorenz) Lacan developed his theory of the ego and the mirror.[4] It is worth quoting Lacan from several different points in his classic offering, "The Mirror Stage as Formative of the I Function" ([1949] 2002), to encounter the inaugural moment this concept was proffered, and to get a feel for the seriousness of the rhetorical style and the ambition of its conceptual reach.

To set the stage: the "development" referred to in the second quotation below is that of the human infant, marked by "a specific prematurity of birth," who at around six months of age begins a romance with himself by becoming enamored of his image in the mirror. This is an exteriorized image the primary caregiver (usually the mother) speaks to and encourages—"Look at you! There you are!"—and with which the young child begins to identify. Thus "identity" is, in its origin, "other," as the child comes to relate to himself as "that" image which is outside. "It suffices," Lacan writes,

> to understand the mirror stage ... *as an identification* in the full sense analysis gives to the term: namely, the transformation that takes place in the subject when he assumes an image—an image that is seemingly predestined to have an effect at this phase, as witnessed by the use in analytic theory of antiquity's term, "imago." (76)

And, later in the same paper he writes:

> This development is experienced as a temporal dialectic that decisively projects the individual's formation into history: the mirror stage is a drama whose internal pressure pushes precipitously from insufficiency to anticipation—and, for the subject caught up in the lure of spatial

---

[3] The psychoanalytic concept of "character" is more complex than I have indicated here. Certainly character extends beyond the ego to include a host of other aspects—temperament, sexuality, defensive structure, and moral conscience—that involve the entire personality.

[4] Roudinesco (2003) details Lacan's debt to Henri Wallon, who coined the term "mirror test" in 1931.

identification, turns out fantasies that proceed from a fragmented image of the body to what I will call an "orthopedic" form of totality—and to its final donned armor of an alienating identity that will mark his entire mental development with its rigid structure. Thus, the shattering of the *Innenwelt* to *Umwelt* circle gives rise to an inexhaustible squaring of the ego's audits. (78)

Whether we take the mirror stage literally, as a stage of development, or take it rather as the foundational myth of the psychoanalytic ego, is no matter. The key claims Lacan makes can be summarized as follows:

1. The ego in its essence is an unstable narcissistic structure, a scaffolding of alienating identifications with highly cathected others (i.e., mirror-self, mother, father, siblings, etc.). (We might note, in passing, the resonances with Winnicott's concept of the False Self.)
2. These identifications are transformative and set the subject on a perpetual, anticipatory quest for mastery, self-sufficiency, a *Gestalt* totality.
3. Thus, identification is a "lure," based upon the specular ("special") capture of the ego by the other. The external image is in tension with the subject's dispersed, bodily experience.
4. The ego's method is comparative, as it attempts to "square" (i.e., reconcile) its fantasmatic image of itself with the others it encounters in the world. This is what Lacan means by the "inexhaustible squaring of the ego's audits": we tend to "see ourselves in the other," and measure the other on the basis of ourselves. Aggressivity and rivalry are inherent potentials, background properties that condition the ego's alertness, wariness of difference, and longing for similarity.[5]

Here is an example of the ego's comparative method. In his discussion of a clinical case described by Ernst Kris, Lacan ([1954] 2002) writes: "For insofar as he [Kris] has concretely indicated what his approach consists of, we clearly see that the analysis of the subject's *behavior patterns*[6] amounts

---

[5] A rarely noted connection here is to the work of the American pragmatist and sociologist George Herbert Mead (whom, as far as I know, Lacan never read). Mead wrote of the "self": "The self, as that which can be an object to itself, is essentially a social structure, and it arises out of social experience" (1934, 140). For Mead, the self (i.e., the ego) is tied to the other through linguistic communication, and so can take itself as an object by identifying with the other's position within the social interaction. Rivalry, envy, aggression, and psychoanalytically conceived motivations in general, were not a part of Mead's pragmatic, in-the-world approach.

[6] This phrase is in the original English in Lacan's text.

to inscribing his behavior in the analyst's patterns" (331). That is, Kris sees and interprets the patient's "behavior patterns" from his, Kris's, own never-neutral perspective. Kris, like all of us, "sees himself in the other."

## Tversky and Kahneman: Cognitive Bias and the "Ego's Audits"

Lacan's insight contained in the mirror stage is of great importance. Much of this book stands squarely on its theoretical and clinical implications regarding the ego, the analyst-as-person, and the analyst's desiring position. But how do the assertions I just summarized line up with our clinical experience? And do scholars who approach the same set of issues from other non-psychoanalytic perspectives support these claims? Regarding clinical experience, subsequent chapters will speak to this question. Here I want to link up Lacan's formulations on the ego with the groundbreaking research on cognitive bias by psychologists Daniel Kahneman and Amos Tversky (described in Kahneman's *Thinking, Fast and Slow*, 2011).[7] Kahneman and Tversky studied the activity of human judgment—a cherished ego function—under a variety of uncertain conditions and therein they discovered different kinds of bias. The array of biases Kahneman and Tversky describe are precisely the kinds of shoring up to which Lacan alerts psychoanalysts. As I already mentioned, Lacan's opaque reference to the "ego's audits" speaks to the myriad ways in which the ego seeks its own satisfaction, its own support, as it forever tries to fortify its borders.

One can locate accounts of the Imaginary resister in numerous places in Lacan's work, especially in the 1950s. A particularly apposite commentary can be found in Seminar III. There one finds an extended critique of "psychology" and its illusory connection to psychoanalysis.[8] In his discussion of Karl Jaspers's classic text, *General Psychopathology*, Lacan describes features of the *relation of understanding* that are entirely consonant with the findings of Kahneman and Tversky. In highlighting key aspects of their work

---

[7] Kahneman won the Nobel Prize in Economics for this work in 2002. Tversky died in 1996. Michael Lewis's book, *The Undoing Project: A Friendship That Changed Our Minds* (2016), chronicles their relationship, their key discoveries, and their wide influence on a variety of human endeavors, from economics, to medical diagnosis, to the assessment of baseball players.
[8] This radical claim—that psychoanalysis is about another level of human experience than the psychological—has been especially influential on French psychoanalysts for two generations, including André Green, among others.

on cognitive bias, I will interpose observations from Lacan to demonstrate this consonance.[9]

In their classic and copiously cited paper, "Judgment under Uncertainty: Heuristics and Biases," published in *Science* in 1974, Tversky and Kahneman describe three basic types of bias (based on numerous studies both in their lab and published by other psychologists):

1. *Representativeness*—the degree to which A resembles B according to specific features. The question subjects were asked took the form, "Is a specific A among the class of Bs?" For example, subjects were asked if person A with specific characteristics was more likely to be an engineer or a librarian. Subjects routinely *overestimated* the predictive power of representativeness. The problem here is that subjects tended to ignore the probability of outcomes (what is known as *prior probability*). For example, engineers are more common in the population than librarians, but this fact was minimized by most subjects who were asked to predict whether person A's occupation was one or the other. Here we have a bias that Lacan described in his critique of Kris: the method of "pattern recognition"—representativeness—as a basis from which the psychoanalyst may come to understand and intervene. In Seminar III, Lacan gives another example of this kind of bias in discussing Jaspers's ideas.

> Understanding is evoked only as an ideal relation. As soon as one tries to get close to it, it becomes, properly speaking, ungraspable. The examples that Jaspers takes as the most important—his reference points, with which he very quickly and inevitably confuses the notion [of understanding] itself—are ideal references. But what is striking is that in his own text he cannot, despite all the hard work he puts into sustaining this mirage, avoid giving precisely the examples that have always been refuted by the facts. For example, since suicide demonstrates a tendency towards decline, towards death, it seems that each and every one of us could say—but only if one sets out to get us to say it—that it more readily takes place at the decline of nature, that is, during autumn.

---

[9] The clinical implications of these findings and observations for the psychoanalyst's assessments as she struggles to understand her patients are, I believe, substantial. Clinical axioms such as listening with evenly suspended attention (Freud), approaching each session without memory and desire (Bion), not identifying with the subject supposed to know (Lacan), inhabiting the analyst's lacking position (Chapter 5, this volume)—all point the analyst in a direction away from bias, away from the auditing methods of the ego. Notably, each of these axioms can become ossified and therefore a site of resistance in the analyst.

Yet it has been known for a long time that many more people commit suicide in spring. That is neither more nor less understandable. Surprise at their being more suicides in spring than autumn can only be based on this inconsistent mirage called the relation of understanding—as if there were anything that could ever be grasped in this order! ([1955] 1993, 6–7)

Here the relation of understanding (which, obviously, is a misunderstanding) is based on the representativeness bias, a *formal similarity*—in this case, *decline*—that is belied by the facts.

Importantly, there are several sub-instances of the representativeness bias (e.g., insensitivity to sample size, misconceptions about chance and regression, illusion of validity, etc.) about which I will not go into detail here.

2. *Availability of instances.* Often people must determine what kind of event or person they are encountering. We routinely appeal to seemingly similar instances that can be easily brought to mind, as in, "this reminds me of that," or "he reminds me of him." *Ease of retrieval* is confused with *frequency* of a given kind of event. *Near-term bias*, relying on a recent event to understand a present one, and *saliency bias*, relying on a particularly impactful or memorable event (which is often near-term), are two common subtypes of *availability bias*. The ubiquity of *false correlation* is another, related bias in this class of biases. For example, in a study of correlation bias in medical diagnosis, Tversky and Kahneman observe: "The illusory correlation effect was extremely resistant to contradictory data. It persisted even when the correlation between symptom and diagnosis was actually negative, and it prevented the judges from detecting relationships that were in fact present" (1974, 1128).

The stickiness of bias—its resistance to contrary evidence—is not limited to false correlations. First impressions, among other biases, are remarkably resistant to contrary evidence, and a large number of people respond to such evidence by *reinforcing* these first impressions (Rabin 1998). Again, we have here clear support for the self-reinforcing nature of ego functioning, in this case the use of cognition and so-called "rational" judgment.

Lacan observed that correlation can easily be read as causation in the example of a child being hit and his crying in response:

When you give a child a smack, well! It's understandable that he cries—without anybody's reflecting that it's not at all obligatory that he should cry ... When one gets a smack there are many other ways of responding than by crying. One can return it in kind, or else turn the other cheek, or one can also say—Hit me, but listen! A great variety of possibilities offer themselves. ([1955] 1993, 15)

3. *Anchoring*. This idea is sometimes known as *reference level*. Here I will quote Tversky and Kahneman:

> In many situations, people make estimates by starting from an initial value that is adjusted to yield the final answer. The initial value, or starting point, may be suggested by the formulation of the problem, or it may be the result of the partial computation. In either case, adjustments are typically insufficient. That is, different starting points yield different estimates, which are biased toward the initial values. We call this phenomenon anchoring. (1974, 1128)

While this particular bias is complex and has many far-reaching implications (including, most famously, the nature of happiness or contentment itself, about which Kahneman has written extensively), for my purposes the issue is one of assuming something to be the case *so that* one can make sense of the clinical sequence or interaction.

Again, prefiguring this work on bias, Lacan describes the basic problem with the *relation of understanding*:

> The major progress in psychiatry since the introduction of this movement of investigation called psychoanalysis has consisted ... in restoring meaning to the chain of phenomena. This is not false in itself. But what is false is to imagine the sense in question is what we understand. What we are supposed to have learned, once again, as is thought everywhere in medical quarters, the expression of psychiatrist's *sensus commune*, is to understand patients. This is a pure mirage.
> The notion of understanding has a very clear meaning. It's a source that, under the name of *relation of understanding*, Jaspers has made the pivot of all so-called general psychopathology. *It consists in thinking that some things are self-evident*, that, for example, when someone is sad it's because he doesn't have what his heart desires. Nothing could be more false—there are people who have all their heart desires and are still sad. Sadness is a passion of quite another color. I would like to insist on this. ([1955] 1993, 6; second emphasis added)

Anchoring points or reference levels are precisely those points from which one begins to "make sense" of a phenomenon; we assume, as Lacan observes, that these starting points are, in fact, beginnings, and are, therefore, self-evident.[10]

We will have ample time to consider the clinical implications of the Imaginary register, the ego, narcissism, and bias. For now, I want to emphasize the nature of the ego as wavering, even frightened; the nature of the psychoanalyst's ego is no different.[11] If we think again about the strangerness that inheres in the psychoanalytic encounter, as I described in Chapter 2, it becomes perhaps clearer why the analyst would struggle with her status, her picture of herself, and naturally work to "square" her experience by minimizing difference and reducing confusion or mystery. The ubiquity of bias speaks to this fundamentally wavering aspect, the automatic movement toward the perpetual shoring up of the ego that uncertainty motivates. Another way to make this point is to say that the analyst lives with a perpetual push within herself to *reproduce* herself in the other in order to make herself feel safer.[12]

## An Illustration from a Consultation

Here is an example from a clinical supervision of the representativeness bias. An analyst, in consultation with me, struggled with his various worries about his patient, especially when the patient expressed despair about the condition of his life, its various tasks and burdens. A successful professional and father of two teenage children, the patient foregrounded his complaints and a deep sense of his own ineffectiveness. When he did so, the analyst often felt, wrongly in my view, that the patient *really was* in a very bad way. There was ample evidence that the patient responded in a more unusual, alive, and open fashion when the analyst did not express, or even silently experience, worry about the patient based on what he was saying to the analyst at that moment.

---

[10] Hirsch, in his *Coasting in the Countertransference*, writes: "The gathering of analytic material becomes a self-fulfilling prophesy—the data are determined by the questions we are predisposed to ask. Analysts look at the environment for identifiable patterns, and perceptions are organized around these configurations" (2008, 115).

[11] See Donald Moss's (2016) "The Insane Look of the Bewildered, Half-Broken Animal," for an extended, brilliant, and multidimensional take on this very issue.

[12] Akerlof's (1970) work on asymmetric information is another angle on the same set of issues. Akerlof showed that if consumers of a product—for example, used cars—have less information about a potential purchase than the seller, the consumer will discount the value of the car. In other words, out of a self-protective anxiety—a quest for safety—the true market value of the car is distorted. Akerlof showed that in such circumstances the entire used car market would gradually fall apart.

In one session, the analyst tells me, the patient described feeling "all alone. As if he's in a cage."

But this recitation immediately brings the analyst up short: "That's funny," he says to me. "The patient didn't say 'cage'. He said, 'cave'. As if he's in a 'cave'."

"A cave you can walk out of," I say.

"Right. Yes. And a cage you can't."

"What's the 'yes' about?"

"It brings home to me how I'm so much more negative about his prospects than he is about himself. He has more room to maneuver than I imagine he does."

We can say, on one level, that here the analyst is having difficulty with a specific kind of bias, the *representativeness* bias: he believes that the patient is in great trouble because the patient describes features of his life that appear to signify a greatly troubled life. And, obviously, the analyst's personal history, the details of which I know very little, must serve to invest "worrying" or "complaining" with a particular significance. In such a case, the potential of the speech relation for new possibilities is greatly reduced, even collapsed. My task as a consultant is to help the analyst see the ways in which he is caught in an Imaginary identification with aspects of the patient's ego-self, an identification that precludes his hearing the potentialities in the patient's speech for other arrangements. Here, the analyst's parapraxis—"cage" for "cave"—is precisely what brings this struggle into the clearing of the now-and-the-next (the now-and-the-next of the consultation; and also, *après-coup*, of the analysis itself) so that an important *difference* between himself and his patient can be *felt*. This felt difference may then lead the analyst to consider more thoroughly this question of the "cage." "Cage" has a chance to become that "stitch-word" (Litowitz 2014) which calls for translation, further expression, further thought. Through this translation process the analyst may come to appreciate more deeply his desire (i.e., fear, anxiety, fantasy, hope) in relation to his patient, as well as being more open to further possibilities. In this case, a few weeks later, the analyst, in consultation, said that the patient was being "cagey"—yet another translation, furthering the analyst's capacity for emergent thought, a key aspect of his desire as an analyst.

## The Closural Nature of Narrative

The biases that I have discussed in this chapter are essentially ways in which the subject, including the psychoanalyst, creates a narrative to give shape to and make sense of enigmatic experience—the so-called judgment under uncertainty. Such enigmatic experience runs the gamut from the totality of one's life (i.e., "Why am I here?" "What am I to do?") to the specifics of a given situation ("What is going on now?"). If psychoanalysis is fundamentally structured by the speech-relation, it may surprise some readers to hear that clinical psychoanalysis is not, at least centrally, work that involves narrative. The formations and realizations of the unconscious within the psychoanalytic moment as it is experienced by analyst and analysand are not at all about a hidden possession now revealed, an ontic thing, a substance finally disclosed, let alone an explanatory narrative such as an organized "unconscious phantasy," "role-relationship model," or "script." These various forms of narratives have nothing to do with psychoanalytic experience as it is unfolding in the now-and-the-next of the work. The difference between a narrative and a psychoanalysis is one of kind—they are different species.

Narrative descriptions have great value for the psychoanalyst when presenting a case to colleagues or constructing a clinical vignette as part of an original piece of psychoanalytic writing. These extra-clinical functions of narrative tend to have identifiable features. They are not simply vehicles for the faithful representation of clinical facts. They are at the same time pieces of rhetoric meant to persuade. This is especially true for the typical clinical case published in the literature. From Freud and Breuer's (1895) *Studies in Hysteria* onward, the trajectory of the psychoanalytic case vignette often takes a familiar form, which is, roughly speaking, that of the short story:

*It is a dark and stormy night: the protagonist is in some kind of trouble.*

There's a problem: the patient is difficult, or the analyst is confused.

*Then something happens in which the character acts blindly and the stakes are raised.*

There's an enactment, a mutually created resistance, an impasse. The patient, and especially the analyst, are operating in the dark. This part usually lasts a while.

*Finally, a veil is lifted as our hero gets new information, experiences an illumination, often of the painful variety.*

After much hand-wringing and internal struggle, the analyst understands something hitherto not seen, not understood. (slightly amended from Wilson 2016)

The fictional short story usually ends there, with the painful illumination.[13] But the analytic short story must continue because *something new and*

---

[13] Charles Baxter writes: "The logic of unveiling has become the dominant mode in Anglo-American writing, certainly in fiction, particularly short stories. We watch

*different* ought to occur. And so, in possession of new insight, the analyst changes her position. This change has felicitous effects on the patient and the entire analysis. *Night, in other words, has turned to day.* If everything is not right with the world, things at least are better in the analysis.

Dhipthi Mulligan, in an illuminating paper called "The Storied Analyst: Desire and Persuasion in the Clinical Vignette" (2017), details the ways in which both the representational requirements and rhetorical features of the vignette are always at work in its telling. Mulligan extends the point that the typical case history is plot-structured like a short story to show that elements of both detective fiction and the epic poem are constitutive of it: *If at one time blind because of seemingly insuperable obstacles, now, with great effort and perseverance, we can see.* The writer-analyst is not only representing her work in the vignette (i.e., what "really happened"), she is also a character in the story that she is telling. By depicting the analyst as both a clever sleuth and a determined healer, the reader is invited to admire (and identify with) the analyst qua analyst, while perhaps not appreciating that the machinery of rhetorical persuasion is being used to effect this admiration and identification.

It is common for all analysts, at various points in a psychoanalytic treatment, to see ourselves in precisely these ways: in the face of obstacles both obscure and obvious, the analyst is a determined and at times clever healer who pieces together new ways of understanding and explaining the patient's symptoms and predicaments.[14] This picture is not only promoted by our clinical literature, it is an alluring one for the clinical psychoanalyst, who, as I have described in this chapter, is in no way exempt from the vagaries and wavering of the ego and its narcissistic struggles.

This picture of the analyst as both detective and hero may be, perhaps, a temptation that many analysts can abjure, at least for the most part. Narrative, as a kind of psychoanalytic method, is, on the other hand, harder to relinquish. We all want to understand what is before us, to make sense of things, to offer psychoanalytic insight to our patients. And yet, I believe it to be problematic for the analyst to pursue an explicit project of threading together the disparate strands of the patient's life into a kind of explanatory story. Why might this be so? There are at least two reasons. First, to the

---

as a hidden-presence, some secret logic, rises to visibility and serves as the climactic revelation" (2008, 45).

[14] And at times it is of great importance for the analytic work that the analyst makes exactly this effort, whether what is offered as explanation is correct or not. As I described in the case of Joan in Chapter 2, the question is one of less shaping an explanatory story than it is of naming and giving further significance to an event, such as my greeting her in the waiting room.

extent that the analyst identifies herself with the hero/detective image she will tend to invest, and perhaps overly commit to, the explanatory narrative that is being constructed in the analysis. The second reason has to do with the nature of narrative itself: narrative explanations tend to *create their own demands for coherence* as they get built.[15]

In a recently published book, *Conundrums and Predicaments in Psychotherapy and Psychoanalysis: The Clinical Moments Project* (2018), Deborah Harms contributed a vignette in which her patient, Jake, a floundering thirty-something in his sixth year of analysis, suddenly reveals to her that "he had been struggling with a very serious gambling addiction. It had now been over a year since he'd been in a casino, but during his fourteen-year long gambling addiction he had come to owe huge sums of money that necessitated he turn to his parents for loans" (230). Jake's prior complaints about women rejecting him in fact turn out to be about "Lady Luck" letting him down time and again.

Harms's story of Jake is presented, like other cases in the book of which it is a chapter, as highly vexed and troublesome, leaving the analyst confused and upset. The illumination that eventually comes in the typical psychoanalytic success story is said not to arrive here. But if we break free of the constraints of the vignette-as-short-story, in which blindness leads to a freeing insight—the "logic of unveiling"—Harms's case history of Jake raises a fundamental clinical question about the binaries that have marked psychoanalysis from its very beginning: false vs. true, resistance vs. freedom of association, repetition vs. new material, discovery vs. creation, darkness vs. light. And Jake's long-withheld revelation about his gambling "addiction" splits these binaries right down the middle, to the analyst's avowed frustration:

> Jake's abrupt confession felt like a punch in the stomach. All these years and all these sessions during which I had worked hard trying to connect the dots to move the analysis along, and yet I had been operating in the dark. The shock of it produced in me anger and a sense of betrayal when I thought about how hard I had struggled to help him with his painful feelings of rejection when he had led me to believe that women were mysteriously and uniformly rejecting him. (213)

The psychoanalyst will feel, at times and in any analysis, overwhelmed, confused, intensely challenged. But in this particular clinical moment it

---

[15] There is a substantial literature on just this issue in contemporary literary studies. See, for example, D. A. Miller's *Narrative and Its Discontents: Problems of Closure in the Traditional Novel* (1981) and *The Novel and the Police* (1988).

is an open question whether a disturbing "darkness" has been revealed or something new and important has emerged in the now-and-the-next. For this author the former possibility takes hold and in disturbing ways. My point is that the analyst's wish to "connect the dots," coupled with hints of the heroic role that, perhaps, allowed her to endure these periods of difficulty, sets her up for the sense of betrayal she now feels. The narrative she had been building regarding Jake's family of origin and his current struggles was so invested with importance that the gambling revelation is not taken as the patient *coming forward with something important and new*, but is instead felt to be, as the author writes, a "punch in the stomach" and a "betrayal." One can imagine a different reaction to this news of Jake's gambling: that it is an illumination, albeit a disturbing kind, but one that suggests that the patient is coming closer to the analyst and is revealing more, not pulling back and revealing less. Harms's case is an example of the ways in which the analyst's dedication to explanation can lead to intense countertransference reactions and conundrums that would not obtain were the analyst less committed to such constructs.

There is not much difference, arguably, between a psychoanalytic narrative that seemingly explains, if partially, the present state of the patient, and, on the other hand, a more rigidly held, paranoid explanation.[16] This is especially true if the storyteller, the constructor of the narrative, is narcissistically invested in the story he or she is putting together. Harms's case report, like any case report, is filled with clues that we only appreciate in retrospect, *after* the gambling tell: the father was a "cheater," the "hiding" of feelings, "people who hide things," "so that he could sneak away," "using pot made him feel like a criminal," the "chest of coins," "addictive personality." The coherence is built retrospectively. This effort is not without value, but it should not be confused with a psychoanalysis as it is lived. As I wrote earlier in this section, the difference between a narrative and a psychoanalysis is one of kind. If we are too interested in "connecting the dots," then moments of newness, surprise, oddity, confusion, contradiction, and repetition tend to get ignored or devalued. In fact, the psychoanalyst ought to be biased toward narrative's *disruption*, against which something new and different can be appreciated. While we all do this story-building to some extent, it is hazardous to make it the central focus of the analysis.

---

[16] The "logic of unveiling"—in which the surface is viewed with suspicion, and, as Baxter writes, about which "almost everyone has been mistaken"—"leads, fairly quickly, to a fascination with conspiracies" (48).

## Conclusion

The gist of this chapter is that the psychoanalyst ought to be well-versed in, and intimately familiar with, the ways in which he or she can get caught up in the evanescent, the invention or mirage of personal identity—usually packaged in narrative form—precisely so a way out can be found. The analyst is a curator of space; we fight against the forces of closure. As an analyst, I *hope to be dislocated*. And, obviously, one can never relocate to the same place; it is always a different place. In this difference one can live one's desire, a desire that is conditioned by lack and *après-coup*.

# 4

# The Analyst's Desire and the Analyst's Resistance

*What follows is an extended and largely rewritten version of a paper I originally published in 2003. That paper was my first pass through this question of the analyst's desire, the ways in which this desire is ignored or undertheorized, and that this individual and collective scotoma can lead to all kinds of clinical problems, snags, impasses, and iatrogenic trauma.*

Let's go back to 1993, a year that seems, from the glacially slow point of view of psychoanalysis, part of a distant world. There was Lawrence Friedman, brilliant and brash, on a panel at the American Psychoanalytic Association's annual meeting in San Francisco. And there were Owen Renik, Samuel Abrams, Warren Poland, and Jane Kite. Jane was a candidate at the time, a young sapling; the others lofty redwoods in the psychoanalytic forest preserve. Friedman is discussing their panel presentations on the topic, *Resistance: A Reevaluation*.

Since the beginning of psychoanalysis, when Freud the neuroanatomist-cum-dynamic psychologist wrote of psychic energy, its bound and unbound states, its investments (cathexes) and resistances to such investments ... the phenomenon of resistance has had a prideful place in psychoanalytic metapsychology and subsequent clinical theory. The mind, after all, is structured. It has a spatial dimensionality in which psychic agencies take up residence and perform different functions and duties. Like anything else meaningful, in the mind as conceived by Freud, there are boundaries and bulwarks that contain and channel forces such that wishes and fantasies gain or lose value. These boundaries and bulwarks constitute "resistances" within the psyche. At the heart of things, as I will discuss shortly, is the Freudian *Wunsch*, the moment that is the wellspring of the energy with which the mind, as conceived psychoanalytically, organizes itself.

Gradually within psychoanalytic clinical theory, resistance took on special significance. During the psychoanalytic session, Freud noticed the various ways in which patients contested his interpretations and interventions. It takes work on the psychical level, Freud repeatedly asserted, to overcome these objections, just as it takes an activation energy to catalyze a chemical reaction. Eventually, with his reframing of the psychic apparatus into the constituent parts of id, ego, and superego, Freud began what became a several-decades-long examination of unconscious ego defenses that manifested themselves as resistances in the analytic hour. In other words, the analyst does not, in the main, engage patients who willingly and intentionally resist; she encounters patients who *unwittingly* yet inevitably defend and resist. They do this, it was averred, unconsciously. The patient *doesn't know* that he *doesn't want to know* the difficult thing, the unwanted desire, the hateful or shameful feeling, especially in the presence of the analyst. This twofold "not wanting to know" analysts called resistance. The analyst's job, in this view, is to "analyze the patient's resistances," so that they become more familiar to the person who deploys them.

There are subtleties to this clinical approach that I will only briefly address here. For example, Paul Gray's (1994) finely honed technique of "close process monitoring" focused on small shifts in the patient's associations—the changing of topics, for example—and qualities of attention, and quantities of discomfort. In addition to these shifts, Gray spent many pages in his writing on the question of the analyst's authority, especially the analyst's imagined status—to be examined and talked about with the patient—as someone who has the power to declare the patient innocent of all he feels guilty and shameful about. The patient, Gray asserted, is invested in seeing the analyst as a benign and helpful judge. "Own that benignity yourself!" Gray seemed to be saying to his patients. "You don't need me for that. Otherwise, you'll keep searching for someone or other to ease your aching soul until the end of your days." For while, back in the 1980s and 1990s, Gray's technique of pointing out these unconscious (or less than fully conscious) resistances to the patient was extremely popular in American ego psychology. As a way of working clinically, it felt objective, dispassionate, and correct.

Well, there are not a few problems with this perspective, especially as it relates to clinical work, and psychoanalytic writing over the last thirty years has, at least in some circles, attempted to address, even redress, these problems. The first issue is that such a view, if fully embraced, places the analyst in a position of authority that resists being analyzed, as the analyst imagines herself to be outside of the analytic field, as if she were not part of an ongoing process and engagement. She is, in this picture, dispassionately and objectively pointing out to the patient the ways in which the patient doesn't want to know something (the way, as we were taught as candidates, to show the patient how his "mind works"). It is not that the analyst already knows this something; it's more that the analyst can sense the patient's wish to avoid a further engagement with whatever it is that seems to be the source of his discomfort. As the remarkably clever Irwin Hoffman once wrote: "In trying so hard to stay out of it, we [analysts] can really *be* 'out of it'" (1996, 106, emphasis in original).

Though Gray was mindful of the problem of the analyst's authority, there is no way for the analyst to be outside of that problematic, no matter how carefully this authority is "analyzed." It's the same problem as with the analysis of transference: the problem of authority is simply pushed one step further back, with an infinite regress just around the corner. How, in other words, does the analyst "analyze" the patient's fantasy of the analyst's being the boss without the analyst continuing to be in that very role? Another problem with "close-process monitoring" is that it risks a kind of claustrophobia in the consulting room. The patient and his discourse are scrutinized for every twist and turn—every turning toward and twisting away—and there sits the analyst, ever-present with her "evenly-hovering attention." The effect is similar to the practice of "too-close reading" that literary scholar D. A. Miller (2013) writes about: the desire on the reader's part to get as close as possible to the "mother" text, inside it, where all its fleshy wrinkles and ink stains are right there before you, super-present. And, as I already said in quoting Hoffman, who decides what constitutes these changes, these movements, these stains and mistakes, these "resistances"? Answer: the psychoanalyst. The analyst assumes not only a position of authority in relation to her patient but also a position safely off the playing field (like a football coach on the sidelines). The key point is this: if the analyst "observes" that the patient has changed topics—"you were talking about this difficult phone call with your mother, and then your voice trailed off"—then the analyst has herself revealed a near-term desire: that the patient continue to talk about that which he has just allegedly veered away from: "Talk more about your mother!" Even or perhaps especially with an analytic technique so carefully honed to the patient's every move, so carefully and closely observant, we can see a shrouded yet no less intense analytic desire at work.

It was at this moment in the history of ego psychology within American psychoanalysis that Friedman made his crucial intervention. The four panel participants about whom Friedman commented described intimate engagements with their analysands—engagements that involved struggle, negotiation, subtle coercion and conflict, and resolution. Renik desired that patients "work" effectively on their problems. Poland wanted an experience in which the analysand felt "present-tense" to him; he wished for the patient to "come alive" in his experience of himself and his analyst. Abrams was concerned with the patient's fantasy of the analyst's authority (not unlike Gray). He believed that the proper focus of analytic investigation was the patient's assumption that a hierarchy existed between them. One way or another, by hook or by crook, these cases resolved satisfactorily, or so each panelist reported.

In fact, as I described in Chapter 3, there is almost always a positive resolution in a psychoanalytic case report. But not with the fourth analyst, Jane Kite, whom Friedman applauded most generously. At that time Kite was a candidate in search of a control case, and she grappled straightforwardly with her desire for the new analytic patient she "needed." Candidates need patients in analysis, otherwise they will not graduate. This one didn't work out, as I recall. Friedman pointed out that Kite was honest about her struggle to accommodate her wish to have a patient in analysis in light of the reluctance of her current prospect. There it was in all of its crystalline clarity: the analyst's desire—when congealed into a wish with a clear aim and object—and the patient's "resistance" to recognizing or acceding to this desire are coupled, conjoined. To Friedman's ear, the other analysts, however senior, venerated, and brilliant, were less aware that they wanted something from their patients and of what they wanted from their patients. They naturalized their desire, as each assumed that his desire for a particular analytic engagement and process was inherent in psychoanalysis itself, in the technical application of theoretical principles, and in the goals of analysis however defined. The deeply held and deeply personal desires of these analysts for particular experiences with their patients—working on problems, coming alive in the analytic relationship, and realizing the inhibiting nature of idealization—became clothed in essentialist notions of the psychoanalytic process.

One is reminded of Lacan's statement of the issue in his Ethics seminar:

> The deep dissatisfaction we find in every psychology—including the one we have founded thanks to psychoanalysis—derives from the fact that it is nothing more than a mask, and sometimes even an alibi, of the effort to focus on the problem of our own action—something that is the essence and very foundation of all ethical reflection. (1992, 19)

Friedman pulled off the mask, he gave a lie to the analyst's alibi that she is rightly proceeding according to the ways a given psychoanalytic community says analysis ought to be done, according to a given theory, and with a correct technical approach. Human desire, Friedman tells us, is never absent from human endeavor. There is no such thing as "natural" work, devoid of human intention and action. "Professional wishes are no less wishes," Friedman writes. "Analysis is a real-world activity. Analysts want to analyze. They like to watch patients in analysis. They want patients to accomplish analytic goals" (1993, 19). But even this description of the analyst's activity is a little too anodyne, as Friedman pulls his punches ever so slightly. Here is Friedman again, in another part of his discussion, more forceful and direct: "There's a demand for work here ... a bending of purpose, a conflict of wills, a verdict of satisfactoriness. The analyst is not just a facilitator; he is a taskmaster and judge" (1993, 13). Yes, a demand, a conflict, a verdict. That captures things better. Resistance has no meaning unless there is a force pushing against it. Resistance, Friedman concludes, is as much about the analyst and his or her wishes as it is about the analysand and his or her conflicts.

The concept of resistance has fallen into disuse for any number of reasons, some valid, and others perhaps not so much. But back when resistance was still a going concern as a meaningful clinical concept, analysts often discussed the stickiness, if not the ubiquity, of *narcissistic* resistances. In the terms used in Chapter 3, narcissistic resistances have to do with the stickiness of bias, a self-protective effort to maintain one's position, one's self-esteem, one's identity in the face of uncertainly or threat. Kohut (1971) deserves full credit for putting narcissism on the psychoanalytic map as a central aspect of normative psychosocial development, rather than a pathological manifestation of that development gone awry. Lacan, however different he is from Kohut in other respects, also theorized a normal narcissism through his concept of the mirror stage and the structuring of the ego by way of a series of identifications. To the extent that the analyst is invested in particular ways of working animated by specific analytic aims and goals, she is desiring experiences that have a narcissistic basis. These desires are more or less evident to the analysand. No doubt the analyst cannot help but wish for certain kinds of experiences in the analytic process with her patient; working, as I said earlier, has no basis unless one wants to get something from that work. As I will show later in this chapter, the analyst's wish for particular experiences can lead to iatrogenic resistances that have a narcissistic grounding. As a foundational matter, clinical impasses are based on this intersubjective fact: that the analyst is pushing for something she is not getting, and her not getting it is, in turn, getting under her skin. This pushing, and the resistances it causes, can at times be directly traumatic to the patient.

## A Bit of Institutional History and the Question of Colonization

This point of view, adumbrated by Lawrence Friedman, as well as Owen Renik and others—especially at the time I first wrote about the analyst's desire in

2003—was clearly in the minority, at least in San Francisco, where I come from. Renik's cogent and innovative work on the irreducible subjectivity of the analyst had, in the early 1990s, a liberating effect on our community, freeing us from the more arid and formal aspects of ego psychology that tended to constrain and lend moral opprobrium to any action that tested the boundaries of "proper analytic technique." Renik brought Irwin Hoffman, Edgar Levenson, and Haydée Faimberg to San Francisco to talk and teach, thereby invigorating our group with an alive, relationally engaging dialectical spirit—dialectical in the sense that the Other (a patient, a theory, an experience-in-time) can never be appropriated by a master's discourse, which means the analyst is lacking and decentered, thereby forever open to new possibility. Renik, in a series of papers, rewrote the book on analytic action through his ideas about countertransference enactment (1993a, 1993b). Hoffman (1994, 1996) wrote several highly influential papers, including one in which he titled a section heading, "Throwing away the Book"—rather in the rebellious spirit of Becky Sharp's tossing Johnson's *Dictionary* out the carriage window in *Vanity Fair*. Levenson was (and still is) a central voice in interpersonal psychoanalysis; his classic texts, *The Fallacy of Understanding* (1972) and the *Purloined Self* (1991), among several others, remain models of how to do a conceptually rich psychoanalytic scholarship that never loses touch with the deeply human. And Faimberg's (2005) inspired concept of "listening to listening" situated the analyst in a futural, nonproprietary position, leaning into the gap, the openness to what comes next. In San Francisco, new possibilities were in the air, as the seemingly incorrigible constraints of psychoanalytic orthodoxy finally appeared to be loosening.[1]

In retrospect, this liberatory ethos was but a moment in time; it lasted less than a minute or two. Like the intoxicating and sexy summer wind that Sinatra sang about so well, this intersubjective, dialectical spirit came and went. Like a summer romance, it was great fun while it lasted. In its wake—and as if that brief affair never happened—colleagues were devouring the classic papers from the neo-Kleinian school. This is because by 1996 or so the London Kleinian perspective was in sudden ascendance in San Francisco. We were being colonized by a number of Kleinian messengers sent from London—each gifted in her or his own fashion, and every one of them especially good at formulating a case, and developing a narrative of the analysis through a detailed look at clinical process. These messengers—Betty

---

[1] Importantly, Joseph Weiss, who did pathbreaking research on psychotherapeutic process for thirty years at the San Francisco Psychoanalytic Institute—and who was, arguably, the most talented clinician of his generation—was marginalized there by more conservative members for most of his career. See Weiss and Sampson (1986), Weiss (1993).

Joseph, Michael Feldman, Elizabeth Bott-Spillius, John Steiner, and Ronald Britton (all found in Schafer 1997), among others—elaborated the nuances and subtleties of transference/countertransference configurations as expressions of the analysand's unconscious phantasy (always spelled with a "ph-") and of an implicit demand for the analyst to enact a certain role within that phantasy. Transference interpretation was central to this psychoanalytic approach. Overall, one could not help but notice a shift in style and tone, from a rather more freewheeling or less burdened approach to analysis, to something more serious and weighed down; a distinct move from the mixed harmonic registers of major and minor keys that animated a truly analytic and dialectical discourse, to the dominant key of the hegemony of the master. Changes in style and tone are, of course, important. But something more than that had taken place: the analyst's very position was reconceptualized. This crucial change is captured in the following way. That most basic of psychoanalytic questions, "tell me what brings you here," had become, "let *me tell you* what brings you here."

Many of my local colleagues were mesmerized by these analysts and the London Kleinian point of view, and in some ways understandably so—they liked the apparent "depth" and seriousness of the Kleinian approach. There was something that could feel very "experience-near" about it. Others of us were not so smitten. There was a simple reason for our skepticism: the formulation of each case and the narratives that were so brilliantly built were all the same. In other words, a "colonization of the patient's text," to use Antonino Ferro's (2002, 6) apt phrase, was being imposed on the patient. We were still in the domain of the analysis of resistance, but in this case of a particular kind: all patients, it seemed, were struggling with "dependency needs." The patient resisted acknowledging these needs by "projecting" them *into* the analyst, or "pressuring" the analyst to enact something rather than talk to the analyst about whatever it was. Weekends and holiday breaks were thought to be especially significant because dependency and loss of contact with the analyst go together and form a nexus of emotional conflict for the patient. Such was the "pre-comprehensive grid" (Leclaire 1998, 6) that came to us from across the pond.

In retrospect, it is easy to see that the objectivist tendencies in ego psychology—to show the patient how his mind "works"—lived on in the reassuring certainty of the Kleinian approach to clinical practice. The openness that is inherent in a dialectical psychoanalysis, in which the analyst is de-centered and lacking ("irreducibly subjective"), and time is conditioned by *après-coup*, was, as I said a moment ago, vanquished.

There was a second reason not all of us fell under the Kleinian spell: the analyst's desire as a category of inquiry had no theoretical standing in Kleinian clinical theory, either as conveyed to the San Francisco community over the years that they visited us, or in the classic papers we so carefully read. These conceptualizations were all working at the level of the Imaginary register—compelling, certainly, and, as I said, seemingly "deep." But desire was not in the mix, especially from the analyst's side. This is not just a scholastic debate or disagreement between psychoanalytic schools regarding the status of the analyst's desire. No, these are surely distinctions with a real difference, and so have real clinical consequences: *resistance*, and its larger and more serious iteration, the true *clinical impasse*, are a direct result of unrecognized desire, as I will discuss in more detail in a few pages. These impasses are to varying degrees traumatic to the patient.

Is there a connection, perhaps an enduring affiliation, between a desire to colonize a psychoanalytic community and the absence of a theory regarding the analyst's desire? What about the desire of a psychoanalytic group to be so taken over? And further, does an interpretive grid, imposed from without, from analyst onto the patient, involve the colonization of the patient's mind? I will leave these suggestive questions for the reader to ponder as she engages with the remainder of this chapter.

## Desire and Wish

This omission of the desire of the analyst as a theoretical and clinical category worthy of direct inquiry was, and is, highly problematic. My paper, "The Analyst's Desire and the Problem of Narcissistic Resistances," first published in the *Journal of the American Psychoanalytic Association* in 2003, attempted to address these problems. As a starting point, let's say the following: human desire, psychoanalytically conceived, is founded on the absent (usually maternal) object. Desire emerges from this human lack that is constitutive for the child's future development. Desire is close kin to, though it encompasses far more psychic terrain than, Freud's Eros in that it is an irreducible, unconscious force that motivates a generic searching. Make no mistake: I am making an ontological claim—the human person qua human is lacking at the level of being. Desire as necessarily emergent from this lack, this want-in-Being, shares much with Heidegger's concept of *Dasein*: the human being is that being for whom Being is an issue. Being is an issue for us! Obviously. We are enlivened by an inescapable searching, over time, in which experiences accrue and are forged into a totalizing way of structuring reality that includes speaking the absence one lives, as in Freud's exemplary story of his grandson and the *Fort! Da!* This totalizing way of structuring reality becomes constituted, again and again, over time and gradually, by unconscious fantasies and identifications. Desire, in short, is what propels our intentionality and involves our irreducible interest in going on in the world.

Wishes, by contrast, are specific and identifiable manifestations of this more all-encompassing, and therefore all-the-more-hidden, desire. Wishes can be more or less fulfilled and are more or less conscious; desire cannot be fulfilled and is unconscious. Regarding the analyst's desire, it can be seen or glimpsed within the various actions that desire motivates, including why each of us chooses to be an analyst (see Chapter 1), our theoretical persuasions, and the kinds of experiences we want to have with our patients for our own particular reasons. Here we can already sense that unconscious desire and specific wishes may not be so easy to disentangle.[2] Be that as it may, the analyst acts on specific wishes, wishes that may be facilitative or harmful to a specific ongoing analytic process. Whether harmful or helpful, our desires are engaged every moment we do analytic work.

Once upon a time, many analysts—whether ego psychological or Kleinian—claimed that the analyst's wishes for certain experiences represent unresolved neurotic conflict.[3] In this picture, the well-analyzed analyst was "neutral" and her work was burdened, at most, by a few well-understood "blind spots." This state of affairs is an obvious impossibility, because the analyst's wishing is inevitable, her pushing and prodding—however tactful, however gentle—ubiquitous, and her exercising of judgment on the proceedings a central part of her ethical position. The picture of the "well-analyzed" analyst is, then, itself wishful, and points to a fantasy of wholeness, integration, and plentitude, and, at the same time an elision of our basic lacking and desiring state. To believe one is "well-analyzed" is to live in one version of a narcissistic enclosure, precisely what Laplanche warned us about. Human work, as I wrote earlier in this chapter, has no basis unless one wants to get something from that work—unless, to put it plainly, one is lacking at

---

[2] This is an issue I take up in detail in Chapter 6 on Bion and Lacan.
[3] The Lacanian world is no more charitable than these orientations regarding the analyst's various untoward desires and countertransference intrusions. But with Lacan's banishment from the International Psychoanalytic Association (IPA) in 1964, his influence took a strange turn and in many parts of the analytic universe it is basically nonexistent (except as ramified through the work of André Green, Jean Laplanche, and others). There exists a vast and faction-ridden Lacanian school outside of the IPA, and Lacanian and post-Lacanian theory continues to have significant influence within the academic world.

the level of being and so is motivated to spend the energy, both physical and psychic, in order to carry out that work.

## Opatow's Intervention

Psychoanalysts have struggled with the proposition—though I believe we might as well call it a fact of human being—that our cherished "rationality" is shot through with self-interest. Aristotle argued that what makes human beings human is their capacity for rational activity, the putting to use of practical reason in the undertaking of various goal-directed actions. It's a justifiably famous argument, and one that psychoanalysis, it would seem, put to rest certainly by the time Freud wrote "On Narcissism: An Introduction" in 1914. But many psychoanalysts, starting with Freud, have cherished rationality, and with the advent of ego psychology it appeared, for a time, that psychoanalysis had saved the Cartesian subject (the subject who arrives at certainty through doubt) from a narcissism that tilts the ego and distorts reality, withdraws from objects and the clarity of a rightly perceived world. As Freud's structural model gained in prominence, the narcissistic basis of the ego was deemphasized. American ego psychologists (Hartmann, for one) tended to highlight the ego's rational capacities, and they insisted on a distinction between the ego and the self. Hartmann (1950) writes: "It therefore will be clarifying if we define narcissism as the libidinal cathexis not of the ego but of the self" (85). Why would Hartmann want to make this separation? Because in doing so the ego is more or less cleansed of narcissistic needs and the influences of the drives (sex and aggression). With the advent of the structural model, the theoretical status of the ego changed: it was now conceptualized as a *set of functions* that gained an autonomy from the internal, thereby allowing it, so the Hartmannian story went, to adapt healthily to the world relatively unburdened by internal exigencies and pressures.

When I read Barry Opatow's papers on metapsychology over twenty years ago now, I felt I had found a theoretical understanding that supported what I had been observing clinically and also grasped from Lacan: that more essential than the gratifications we might hope for in doing analytic work is *the wishfulness inherent in our being thinking and feeling persons.* The irreducibility of the analyst's desire starts there. Opatow's paper, "The Real Unconscious: Psychoanalysis as a Theory of Consciousness" (1997), was especially helpful to me in digging deeper into the relations between the mind's structuring around wishing and the natural narcissism that emerges from that wishing. Opatow investigates this idea through Freud's concept of hallucinatory wish-fulfillment. For Opatow, the metaphor of hallucinatory wish-fulfillment is foundational for psychoanalytic theory; it is the *original scene* of psychoanalysis. It is also the original scene of the mind as conceptualized psychoanalytically; that is, hallucinating a gratifying image is the genesis of the desiring subject, the subject's origin as subject. This scene, to summarize Freud, unfolds in the following way: in the absence of nourishment, the hungry infant attempts to satisfy itself (or affirm itself) with an image (a memory or sensation) of feeding on the breast. Faced with pain induced by absence, the infant attempts to refind psychically the lost object of satisfaction. Lack generates desire, which manifests itself as a conscious imagining of satisfaction. Opatow writes: "An unconscious wish strives to actualize a scene—to revive it as a conscious event" (873).

Opatow's point is further reaching because he argues that the psychoanalytic postulate that satisfaction can be hallucinated is not limited to a theory of unconscious fantasy. *A hallucinated satisfaction is the foundation of thinking itself.* "What is transferred from unconscious to conscious in the movement up the ordered hierarchy of mind is affirmation per se," Opatow concludes (873). In other words, there is an inherently self-validating aspect to thinking and perceiving. Sound familiar? We are in some of the same territory I covered in Chapter 3, in that Opatow is giving us a picture of the mind, psychoanalytically conceived, that wishes to affirm and reaffirm, to close the circle, to fill the lack that generated the desire at the start. Opatow's work gives us yet another angle on the ego functions of rationality and judgment: there is no such thing as "neutral" thinking. *Thinking is suffused with a distinctly narcissistic, self-aggrandizing desire.* I hope it is clear by this point that I do not mean to imply something pathological in using the term "narcissistic." Thinking is a self-preservative function, and in that very important sense is always already self-serving. In this regard, I am especially appreciative of this quotation from Pontalis (1981):

> Narcissism is not a phase, nor a specific mode of cathexis, it is a position, an insurmountable and permanent component of the human being. Even the most intellectual functions (thinking), the most objective ones (perception of reality), and the forms of behavior which come closest to instinct (eating) are marked by it. (136)

There is nothing to "get over" regarding one's inherent, built-in narcissism. We cannot help but see ourselves in the physical and interpersonal surround of our lives, shoring up our position automatically. These points, obviously, connect directly with the issue of cognitive bias—the squaring the ego's "audits"—that I described in detail in Chapter 3.

## The Analyst's Desire for Particular Experiences

We analysts are always looking for something. I have called this looking "narcissistic" in that we, often enough, want to reestablish ourselves and our felt position as analysts as we work. And what are we looking for, exactly? Obviously, answers to this question are as multiple as there are psychoanalysts and moments of engagement in a clinical hour.

Let's start, again, with Opatow's treatment of Freud's idea of refinding the lost object. Here is one way to put the issue: the analyst unconsciously desires to feel *as if* she is reexperiencing a particular kind of object relationship with analysands. Such a relationship might be with an idea or a theory, not only with a person. The "as if" is extremely important. The analyst is not in fact reexperiencing a past relationship—she is experiencing *this* relationship—but is doing so only in fantasy and in derivative form. The patient's experience of the same clinical moment may be something else altogether. This "refinding" of the object relationship can, and does, take diverse and complex forms. The analyst may attempt to *repeat* moments of relating with patients that unconsciously remind her of pleasurable past relationships. Alternatively, the analyst may wish to *redress* with patients a particularly painful past object relationship or persistent internal conflict (see Jacobs 1991; McLaughlin 1991; Renik 1993b as examples). For instance, an analyst with an emotionally unavailable parent may believe herself to have been the agent of that parent's behavior and may worry, accordingly, about her own omnipotence and destructiveness; that analyst may hope to redress these worries by having emotionally close and intimate relationships with patients. Ella Sharpe (1950) made a related point long ago. She writes of the analyst who suffers from excessive therapeutic zeal—a persistent desire to be helpful and altruistic—in order to manage her unconscious sadism. Such an analyst, uncomfortable with patients who keep their distance, may too quickly and urgently interpret their defensive posture and simply exacerbate problematic aspects of the interaction that instead call for tolerance, patience, and flexible engagement. In a paper I am particularly fond of, Gabbard (2000) speaks to this point in his discussion of the "ungrateful" patient. He writes: "Ungrateful patients, in particular, are likely to make us aware of our unconscious background wish to enact a gratifying object relationship that motivates us to return to the consulting room day after day" (699).

Another way in which analysts can feel stable and "balanced"—on the "right" track—is to feel aligned with a particular theory of mind and clinical process. I have already alluded to how crucially important it is for some analysts (and a significant proportion of a psychoanalytic community) to identify with a given theory or a charismatic emissary of that theory. Several analytic thinkers have noted the importance to the analyst of psychoanalytic theory as a "loved object"—that is, a refinding of a love that has been lost but never given up completely, now reestablished in the analyst's identification with a theoretical model (Almond 1995; Caper 1997; Purcell 2004). The analyst's relationship to theory has many important consequences for her functioning, some of which are clearly necessary for good analytic work to proceed. At a minimum, there is no way to proceed as an analyst without working with an implicit theory of the mind and a view on therapeutic action. Most often, though, if the analyst is "thinking theory" in a clinical hour, she is likely using it as a way to maintain a feeling of independence from difficult internal experiences of whatever valence (boredom, frustration, excitement, hatred, passion, and the like).

We can't do this shoring up and refinding of ourselves alone. We have a natural tendency to want others to recognize our perspectives, ideas, and feelings. This is the basic Hegelian dynamic of two subjects in a dyadic and oscillating relation of lord and bondsman, master and slave. The literature here is vast and spans a couple of centuries. To be brief: *Our desire as human beings is to have our desires recognized by others* (Kojeve 1947; Lacan [1953] 2002; Benjamin 1988; Fukuyama 1992). By "self-aggrandizing desire," then, I don't mean simply a self-centered and solipsistic desire. I have in mind also one's desire for the other's recognition and love. J. H. Smith (1991) puts it well: "Anything anyone does, thinks, or feels is a manifestation of concern for one's being and being-with. Desire at one moment, anxiety at another, arise from a want of being and a want of the other" (92). This "want of being" and "want of the other" gestures toward a *lack* that underwrites all desire, a topic I will discuss in the next chapter.

## Dual Relations: The Analyst's Desire and Resistance

The analyst is always, in part, looking for lost objects, trying to refind herself in the patient and to see herself as an analyst in day-to-day clinical work. The crucial question is how these desires facilitate or hinder a successful analytic process. As I have been suggesting, resistance does not reside "in" the patient;

resistance is fundamentally an intersubjective phenomenon. *The analyst's desire—as it is expressed through specific wishes and demands—engenders resistance when the patient feels forced to recognize it.* Especially during moments of uncertainty or uncomfortable silence or interaction—in which the analyst feels in her bones caught in an enactment with a patient—the analyst is tempted to fall back for defensive purposes on certain cherished identifications with a theory, a supervisor, a colleague, or her analyst. Precisely when we feel lost we want to refind ourselves. Here we are in the by now familiar place of the exercising of judgment under uncertain conditions: bias looms larger in these moments. We "forget" our fundamentally lacking—and therefore mobile, open—position. In our attempts at recovering a (falsely) stable place, we are left less than alert to the patient, to what he might be experiencing and, especially, what he is expressing or struggling to express. These resistant moments result from "misrecognition," the subtle or not so subtle confusion of self with other.

Some readers may feel that this clinical dynamic of the analyst's imposition of her desire (and the effects of this imposition) is a reassuringly local clinical problem. In my experience, this dynamic runs farther and deeper than is typically recognized, and manifests itself in countless microscopic clinical interactions. The analyst's desire, as manifested in specific wishes, is especially hard to appreciate if one's clinical theory does not include its presence as a—perhaps the—key operator in the analytic process. Any analytic intervention houses within it aspects of the analyst's desire for some kind of response and recognition on the part of the patient.

Under clinical circumstances in which analysts desire too strongly, or too unconsciously, to have specific kinds of experiences with their patients, iatrogenic resistances often result. The impasses that one finds described in clinical psychoanalysis are due, certainly most of the time, to this factor. The patient is put in the alienated position of "needing to deal" with the analyst's desire. Though the analyst's commenting "interpretively" on the patient's response to an intervention may further the analytic dialogue, this is rarely the case because *interpreting the contested interaction by calling the analysand's attention to it only feeds its reinforcement.* In such difficult clinical circumstances, which are more common than is usually acknowledged, there can be no clear way out. A crucially important aspect of these narcissistically based resistances is that, from a logical point of view, the dynamics asserted to be going on in the patient can just as easily be asserted to be going on in the analyst. Lacan called this way of interacting a "dual relation." *Dual relations are inherently reversible.* Both analyst and patient want the other to recognize their desire. When caught in a dual relationship, it is often difficult to figure out what is what; confusion results.

Let's return now to the London Kleinians. They tend to provide telling clinical examples that demonstrate precisely this issue. Joseph, in her classic paper "A Clinical Contribution to the Analysis of Perversion" (1971), describes an interaction with her patient, Mr. B, that illustrates the difficulties posed by the analyst's desire for specific clinical experiences and the reversible nature of dual relations. Joseph's focus on the patient's emotional contact, or lack thereof, with the analyst is central to her clinical point of view. Her analytic desire, in other words, is trained toward this "object"—namely, emotional contact—itself a complex notion. Joseph's ideas on transference, specifically on the totality of transference manifestations in the clinical moment, have been hugely influential; everything the patient says or does has immediate transference meaning and "bends" the analytic relationship in ways that are unconsciously both gratifying and necessary for the patient. As we will see in a moment, the role of the analyst's desire has no independent theoretical standing in Joseph's conceptualization of the analytic encounter. What we have, instead, is the imposition of an interpretive grid, a powerful one to be sure, but all the more worrisome because of its power, including its power to colonize the patient's text.

Joseph's focus on emotional contact and the totality of the transference leads her to consider patients' reactions to weekends and holidays—periods of time away from the analyst—as important topics for analytic consideration. In the complex case of Mr. B, Joseph describes a man with a narcissistic character structure and baroque sexual practices. Let's assume that, as with all published clinical material, the analyst's understanding of the case has a privileged status, and it is to her credit that Joseph provides us with enough information to allow alternative readings of it. Mr. B, well into his analysis, gets married over a summer holiday. Upon his return, a number of complicated interactions ensue between him and his analyst, including, among other things, an elaborate dream. I want to focus on one specific aspect of Joseph's discussion. Mr. B tells his analyst that he was frightened to let her know about his recent marriage. He was worried that the analyst, as Joseph writes, "would feel angry and left out, as if he ought not to have put the marriage before the analysis; almost as if he ought to have married the analyst. It becomes clear," Joseph continues, "how much he has projected his own left-out infantile feelings about the holidays onto me, and feels me to be watching, left out and demanding" (445). Joseph does not make "clear" precisely what she said to Mr. B, but she strongly suggests that she interpreted to him his projection of his feeling of dependency onto her. Mr. B is the one who truly feels left out; his worry that the analyst feels left out is defensive, a resistance to the "truth" of the matter.

Yet this is precisely where things get tricky and where, I would argue, confusion can reign in the clinical moment. This is because Joseph wants Mr. B to admit *his* having felt left out over the holiday break. He doesn't acknowledge this, and therefore, in a very real sense, he is not acting in the way she wants him to act. More to the point, Mr. B is not thinking the way his analyst would wish him to think, in that he is not "using" the analyst's interpretations to further his self-understanding. Mr. B, in other words, is not recognizing—satisfying—his analyst's desire. One cannot help but wonder—à la Irwin Hoffman and his influential paper, "The Patient as Interpreter of the Analyst's Experience" (1983)—whether the patient has accurately concluded that the analyst feels the patient *should have missed her*, and, therefore, has understandable concern about thwarting the analyst's wish that he acknowledge feeling "left out" and "watching." In terms of the logic of the interaction, the assertion that the patient misses the analyst and uses omnipotent defenses to ward off his feeling of dependency could be made also about the analyst: that the analyst herself is engaging in omnipotent thinking because she "knows" what is going on with her patient. Further, she wants the patient to relate to her in a particular way that he is not doing, and in that sense she feels "left out," yet she projects this feeling into him. *All the assertions the analyst makes about the patient could be made about the analyst.* The issue is not whether this reading is correct. The issue is that in a dual relation there is always an alternative, symmetrical reading and that it is impossible to know which of the two readings is correct. For any patient in such a situation, the confusion and torment that can result cannot be gainsaid; the patient is left not knowing up from down. The reason any patient in such a bind can feel torment is because of the analyst's transferential authority and potential exercise of power in light of this authority. In these moments, a radical kind of misrecognition holds sway, as the analytic space is collapsed. Jessica Benjamin (2004) has written extensively, and quite brilliantly, on this very phenomenon, a clinical interaction that she calls "doer and done-to."

Let's compare Joseph's approach to that reported by Gabbard (2000). Gabbard, in the case of Mr. F, wants Mr. F's recognition for his (Gabbard's) "dutiful and steadfast service" to him (698). Gabbard's desire, grasped by his perspicacious patient, contributes to a resistance. Gabbard writes about his desire in this way:

> The child's desire for a long-denied gratitude may in adulthood take the form of a yearning to be appreciated by one's patients, even to the point of encouraging expressions of gratitude that are at odds with the patient's

best interests. In such a situation, the analyst's need for gratitude may become apparent to the patient, who then feels that the analytic setting is being subverted to address the analyst's needs. (700)

Gabbard then reflects on how his patient reacted to his (Gabbard's) desire for recognition:

> Repeating the scenario that occurred with his parents, he sensed that I wanted him to fall in line with my expectations, and he derived great pleasure from digging in his heels and defeating me. I had failed to appreciate that he was trying to communicate to me that he was doing the analysis in the way he had to do it, and that my failure fed his own developmental difficulties in feeling appreciative. (705)

Gabbard attributes the turnaround in the case of Mr. F to three factors: (1) Gabbard's resilience in the face of his patient's attacks, (2) his recognition of what he calls "the two-person nature of the problem. My awareness that my countertransference resentment was contributing to the impasse" (710), and (3) successful interpretation of the patient's internal conflict. No doubt Gabbard is correct. However, I would argue that the second factor, Gabbard's acknowledgment of his countertransference resentment, is what allowed the stalemate to yield because the battle, at that point, was no longer joined. And with the battle no longer joined, there was, as Gabbard describes, space for both him and Mr. F to consider Mr. F's conflicts and "symbolize his experience." An additional point worth reiterating, and one that Gabbard acknowledges though in my estimation underemphasizes, is the fact that his desire for gratitude—not simply his resentment of his patient's ingratitude—contributed to, and in important ways engendered, Mr. F's resistance, the digging in of his heels. You can't resent a patient's being ungrateful unless you wanted his expression of gratitude to begin with.

In light of this comparison between the clinical offerings of Joseph and Gabbard, I ask the following question: At the level of the resistance as experienced by the patient in the clinical moment, is there a difference between an analyst whose desire is expressed through a model of the mind and a clinical technique that emerges from that model (Joseph), and an analyst whose desire is manifested in the wish for a gratifying object relationship based on a persistent conflict from the analyst's past (Gabbard)? It seems to me our conventional answer to this question is that the latter is much more suspect, because it implies that the analyst has more self-analytic work to do. Gabbard, so this thinking goes, simply needs more analysis himself.

But here is the rub: both analysts are searching for lost objects, just different ones. I believe that the former circumstance is more difficult for the analyst to perceive and self-analyze because her desire is both expressed through and hidden by a clinical technique that, at that particular psychoanalytic moment, is contributing to the resistance. Certainly, at the level at which the resistance is joined, the patient may experience both desires similarly—as the analyst's demand for the patient to respond in a particular way, a demand that puts the patient in an alienated position. The analyst is in a more difficult spot, however, if she cloaks her desire in a theory of technique that she assumes to be true and takes for granted, thereby naturalizing her desire by way of that theory. Gabbard's approach gives the analyst a fighting chance to alter the stickiness, even the tenacity, of the dual relation resistance.

Gabbard takes a measure of his desire, and finds that it had been functioning as a cloak, a shroud, that covers over his patient's subjectivity such that the patient is misrecognized. He finds that his insistence on his patient's expression of gratitude puts his patient in a disturbingly removed, not to say impossible, spot. Here we find ourselves at a moment that is perhaps too common an occurrence in psychoanalytic work, and that has been well-described in our literature over the past twenty or so years. The dual-relation resistance is, as we have seen, a dyadically constructed "field of contest" (as Lacan wrote in his Mirror Stage paper): it is either *you or me, my desire or yours*. There is no breathing room in such a situation, no third term or point of reference that both parties can look to or use to gain perspective on the interaction. In statistics, we know that correlation is not causation; the covariation of two terms is simply that. In order for a reliably valid causal relation to be established an independent variable is needed. In psychoanalysis, it is ethically incumbent upon the analyst to find a way to remove herself from the field of contest. As Jessica Benjamin has emphasized, the question the analyst faces in such moments is one of *surrender*, a yielding. This yielding is not submission, as submission is simply one side of the dual-relation, master–slave dynamic. Surrender entails grabbing hold of one's desire and shifting it through internal work, work that results in a meaningful self-acknowledgment. In so doing the analyst's position is already changing, and the highly viscous analytic field loosens up as things have a chance to flow again.

## Clinical Vignette: Robert

Robert, a divorced man in his late thirties, had struggled in any number of ways through the first year of his analysis. He came for treatment because of periods of crushing despair and hopelessness about the future. Though talented and accomplished in his profession, he was convinced there was something drastically wrong with him. Emerging from a painful divorce some years back, he ruminated in session after session that he would be alone the rest of his life. He was terrified of planning assertively for the future. He had difficulty thinking about his career and the next direction in which he wanted it to go. He desperately wanted to remarry but worried endlessly about being rejected. Like Hamlet or Prufrock, he struggled with key decisions. Letting a woman know he liked her and that he wanted to see her again felt truly like "disturbing the universe." He felt shame at his failed first marriage, as if that failure were an incurable blight on his entire and as yet unlived future.

The youngest of five children, Robert came from a middle-class family where emotions were hard to read and conflicts rarely addressed. Though close to his mother when a young child, he had long since viewed his parents with embarrassment and some shame: they seemed unhappy, scared, and depressed. (He would often note, in a bedraggled tone, that he seemed fated to repeat all of his parents' mistakes, except they had "succeeded" in remaining together "in misery" all these many years—his words—while his marriage had fallen apart.) These feelings drove him, decades ago now, to move far away from the family; he struggled to call or visit them, fearing the feelings of shame, anger, and sadness he often felt when around them. Robert lamented: "My parents don't seem interested in my life, what I'm doing, or what I'm feeling."

Though often hard to put to one side, Robert's sad-sack self-presentation was not so dominant that I was unable to appreciate his sharp mind, wry humor, and his sensitivity to friends and colleagues. He complained about being unattractive, but seemed, to my eye, to down-dress, using a conventional form of "Berkeley casual" to hide his handsome features and rugged build. We had moments of genuine amusement, and at such times the heavy weight of a doomed future lightened some.

I saw Robert soon after becoming a graduate analyst. While not at all wedded to any one theoretical approach, with him I tended to talk "conflict," "inhibition," and "anxiety"—what I think of as "ego psychology" talk. Certainly not wrong—after all, didn't Freud write about inhibitions, symptoms, and anxiety? But, as I have stressed several times over the course of these chapters, talk of "conflict" and the like can feel abstract and distancing; such terms failed to give form to the possibility of Robert sensing something emerging from within that I recognized as his *personal* struggle and pain. Generally speaking, my approach to his problems during this first year of analysis was to examine his conflicts with him (though Robert was often not "with me"), specifically the imagined negative consequences of various actions, should he take them. "How is it, exactly, that you know Kerrie doesn't want to go on another date?" Or, "Oh, I see. So it's easier to think you know the outcome rather than find out. What do you worry will happen?" Such were typical comments I would make to Robert, which he tended to hear not as open-minded questions but as criticisms and subtle prods to be other than he was. Often a few minutes late to sessions, he and I discussed his generally passive stance and the safety he felt in keeping his distance from his friends and me. He tended to view analysis as another painful burden.

As I got to know him I pointed out how he seemed invested in minimizing his talents, that his friends liked him, that Kerrie had told him he was "cute." Being a person well-versed in the art of complaint, Robert had difficulty hearing these comments from me. I often pointed out that he seemed to "get something" out of complaining the way he did. He acknowledged—though by no means owned—that he felt his suffering was "special" and that he deserved special treatment and attention by his family and friends. The nature of "special treatment" remained unclear, and he felt bitterly resentful when friends or family didn't attend to him in this way. We discussed how he expressed his anger through the distance he maintained from people. When possible, I directed his attention to how these issues showed up in our relationship, that is, in the transference. Analysis was a place of suffering too, no different than the rest of his life.

Though Robert appeared to gain much "insight" into his suffering stance toward his life and the world, none of this got us very far. And my approach—pointing out this anxiety and that defense, this hidden strength or that unacknowledged achievement—exacerbated his masochistic sense of analysis; much of the time he felt it an onerous burden. However tactfully and "open-mindedly" I directed Robert's attention to our interaction—and especially to the atmosphere of struggle often between us—he took my observations to be criticisms that he was doing something wrong.

In short, much of the first year or so of analysis felt "contested." What was my contribution to this contest? My subject position with respect to Robert—a perspective gained only in retrospect—could be described as follows: I was a newly graduated analyst looking to build up my analytic caseload. I decided to work with Robert for a "reduced" fee. (This is before I came to the understanding that *all* fees are negotiated, and that the full fee/reduced fee binary is a specious construction.) And I was without supervision. All of these factors contributed to an exaggerated therapeutic zeal on my part, and therapeutic zeal from a particular theoretical point of view.

Within this personal professional context in which I found myself, I identified with the patient's struggles in a number of important ways that only exacerbated my desire somehow to change and "cure" him. For example: Robert regularly told himself to "mellow out" about things, especially about a woman he was dating. He told himself that it's not a big deal whether things worked out or not. As a younger person I myself had struggled with a similar way of thinking regarding a deeply held ambition of mine, and had realized my self-deception only when it was for all practical purposes too late (see Chapter 1). With Robert, I wanted to redress an enduring conflict within myself—or, more accurately, a loss unsuccessfully mourned—with which I had struggled very much alone, and I did so by trying to assure my patient I was "there" for him and would help him avoid the self-deception from which I had suffered.

The ways in which Robert and I discussed this mode of thinking and the anxiety that lay behind it are too complex to characterize adequately. The end result, however, is easy to describe: Robert felt that I was telling him not only to stop thinking this way but to stop *being* this way. Arnold Rothstein's description (1999, 544) of a "sado-narcissistic" enactment captures accurately Robert's and my interaction around this issue. One could say (and many analysts over the years have said just this) that through his tendencies toward masochistic suffering he unconsciously involved me in ways that made him feel further victimized. Perhaps. But that possibility was neither here nor there, because at that point in the analysis, none of this awareness was available to him. What was available to me was an embodied feeling, a visceral sense of "here we are again": once he started his complaints of despair, or his needing to "mellow out and take it slow," I could already feel the enactment occurring, and most any intervention I made that addressed his discourse as defensive, as related to anxiety and worry, led inexorably to his feeling that I was telling him what to do or how to think. I was contributing to a dynamic between us that, at this relatively early point in the analysis, felt contested, stuck, and damaging to him. Without question, I was a "colonizer" of Robert's mind, though I didn't put it that way to myself at that moment. Nor at that time did I fully conceptualize things through the lens of iatrogenic trauma. But the guilt that I felt clearly pointed to this fact: that my way of being with Robert engendered in him a sense of alienation and feeling misrecognized. Importantly, for Robert's part, though he complained with some regularity, he voiced no concerns that the analysis was stuck or that I was contributing to the trouble. His attitude was characteristically passive: "This must be how analysis is."

Well, this is not how analysis "must be." As the stuck, contested feeling was available to me, so were choices to move in other directions, to relinquish previous positions to see what else was possible between us. So I pulled back, and not in a "lick my wounds" kind of way. I quite consciously decided not to interpret the defensive aspects of Robert's pseudo-nonchalance or his complaints of despair. I simply asked him to tell me more about these feelings. I let him know through a variety of questions and an openness in my tone and quality of my presence that I wanted to hear more, not less. Over the next several weeks, seemingly in direct response to this shift in my subjectivity—a shift, that is, in the objects of my analytic desire—Robert gave more full-throated expression to his suffering. And his way of speaking gradually came to have a different aspect. He talked about his despair without massaging it. He had moments of genuinely questioning himself without demanding immediate answers from me or condemning himself for not knowing them. He found himself describing ways in which he orchestrated interpersonal situations so he would feel left out or "dissed." At times, he realized, he "made up" scenarios so, as he said, "I can feel angry and bitter and resentful." I treated all of this with a feeling that was surprising to me. I neither overvalued nor undervalued what he was telling me. I was now settling into being with him without the need to "do anything."

My sense was that Robert's primary wish was to tell me how bad he felt without being thrown off by me—without my desire (or his perception of my desire) getting in the way. As I stopped interpreting the defensive and gratifying aspects of his complaints (from the point of view of intrapsychic conflict, compromise formation, and resistance), he felt I was not implicitly telling him to stop feeling what he was feeling and stop thinking what he was thinking. He now felt that there was more room for him to feel as bad as he wanted to feel and to complain about it as much as he wanted to complain. He was unable, at this point in the analysis, to examine our interaction and his feelings about the analysis without severe superego intrusion. *In my estimation, there was no other way out of this infinite regress than for me to stop contributing to it.* As I removed myself from the field of contest, Robert felt much freer to think about himself. This showed in his ability, perhaps for the first time in our working together, to analyze himself. As he talked about the details of how bad he felt at times, he began to notice he was feeling better. He became more curious about his own thoughts and spoke more freely. He felt more "in control" and less overwhelmed. In short, instead of his feeling that I was implicitly telling him what to do and how to be—forms of ignoring him, as he felt his parents had done repeatedly— he now felt that I did, really and in fact, want to listen to how he was feeling.

Soon after, for the first time in the analysis, he reported a dream:

I'm on some kind of raft with a couple of other people, off shore, not totally at sea, but I'm afraid the waves might overtake us. The raft was made out of concrete, of all things. You'd think it wouldn't float but it floated just fine. We were out there for a purpose; we had a task to do or something. That's all I remember.

He reported this dream in his typically halting manner. We discussed his discomfort in telling me the dream. He had few ideas why he was feeling uncomfortable; he just was. "This is how I've felt a lot in here, though not recently."

Deaf for the moment to his having said that, I replied, "I wonder whether you are worried that if you let your thoughts go about the dream you would be swept out to sea."

He thought about that briefly and said he didn't think so. "Though there was the possibility we might get taken out to sea," he said in a more comfortable tone, "I wasn't all that worried about that." He fell silent and became more halting, and after a while he said he had no more thoughts about the dream.

I then asked him about the piece of floating concrete.

"Yeah, strange huh?"

He was silent again for a bit. "It was about the size of this couch."

I said: "Sounds like the dream has something to do with your thoughts about being here."

In response he got "realistic": "Well, since I am lying on this thing it seems like it was just an easy source of comparison. But I have been feeling stronger recently, more hopeful. Somehow the concrete is related to that feeling, which, I have to say, I'm suspicious of, because it's so foreign to me. Like the sea is my despair, and I feel more confident that I can swim in my depression and handle it without getting swallowed up."

I then asked about the other people who are also holding onto the concrete raft.

"Well, I think it was only one other person, not two. It was a man. We were doing something out there. We were supposed to be there, on a task of some kind ... I guess," he said with surprise, "the other guy sounds like you. It's hard for me to acknowledge that this might be helping me and it's feeling more like we're in this together."

The emergence of the unconscious—Robert's dream—often arises, as it did here, once a dual-relation impasse yields to a more open way of working.

The analytic space is restored. The hothouse of the analytic dyad becomes triangulated. In psychoanalysis, how is this third term established? In a variety of ways, it turns out. But nothing "other" can be heard if the analyst holds his position, his point of view, too dearly.

## Friedman Redux

Robert, obviously halting and tentative in this series of interactions with me, peers from behind his masochistic way of being and begins to see and experience something else, some other, less hopeless way of being. His subject position—as the defeated man with no future—is beginning to change. He talks to me somewhat differently, in a way that is both more his own and more our own. There is a sense of the third now, the dream and our talking, however tenuous and evanescent. When I set aside my conscious agenda, my technique, he begins to find his own faltering voice. And this, in the end, is the sole object of the analyst's desire: that the analysand finds his voice, that he keeps struggling to find it, and thereby steps into fuller possibilities of personal expression and, ultimately, action. I had wanted a certain experience with Robert that was underwritten by a theory of technique (resistance analysis) and my own narcissistic concerns. I first caught onto my use of technique as an expression of my own "stuff" because I saw my approach was not working. Upon further reflection, I realized it was being driven predominantly by an old struggle of mine. Then I saw through my own defensiveness, a defensiveness that amounted to my unwillingness to listen to parts of his mind and heart as reflected in his speech. Who was being defensive? Who was being resistant? We both were, though I was in a position to do something about it. What emerged was a clinical process that was less contested than shared: we were more "in this together." My analytic desire shifted to a different one, more aligned to the patient's interests at the moment. And I would again wonder whether it made any difference to Robert, at the level at which he experienced the resistance, what factors may have driven my contribution to it. If my unresolved conflict was not part of this particular clinical interaction, I still may have contributed just as intensely to the resistant atmosphere by my overall approach of interpreting anxiety and defense.

The gratification I felt from this series of interactions with Robert was substantial. As Friedman said back in 1993, I had reached a "verdict of satisfactoriness." Yet my feeling of satisfaction was not based on any conscious agreement or assent on Robert's part. Nor did I ask him to reflect on why he was feeling more hopeful. It seemed to me that that would be another attempt on my part to claim some therapeutic territory for myself precisely when he was just starting to feel he had a right to some of his own. I felt good simply because I was able to get out of his way enough so he could begin to see himself as an actor in his life, a life that still felt perilous, but a peril brightened by a modicum of hope.

There is no easy resting place in clinical psychoanalysis. With Robert, in subsequent months, my more open and inquiring stance—to which I had become quite attached—itself became a source of resistance. He had retreated again, though perhaps not as far as I feared. The hours had become labored and tiresome. I felt the need to address his retreating more directly, which I did. This time, as though I had enough credit in the psychoanalytic bank, he was better able to talk about his fears of me and others to whom he is close without the degree of suffering that had accompanied such interactions previously. Although Robert was now less brittle, my focusing too frequently, no matter how tactfully, on his anxiety often led to a more contested atmosphere. In the end, my maintaining a relatively flexible stance and not being committed to any one way of being with Robert seemed to be the most important aspect of my working successfully with him. As Kennedy (2000) writes in his illuminating essay on the emergence of subjectivity in psychoanalysis: "I suggest that things take place in various shifting positions between analyst and patient, where the subject opens up or closes down. This shifting becomes the basis for human subjectivity. Becoming a subject involves some sort of opening up; but one cannot ignore the closing down" (884). Clearly in the case of Robert, he and I both were emerging subjects. Any particular position of mine, while possibly salutary at one point in time in contributing to an opening up of the process, could at another contribute to a closing down, to stasis.

While Friedman (1993) is right to emphasize that in psychoanalysis there is a "demand for work ... a bending of purpose, [and] a conflict of wills" (13), we can also say that the analyst's recognition of his demands on the patient, his recognition of the desire and will inherent in the endeavor of analyzing, is the first step toward moving beyond the clinical impasse based on the dual relation resistance. Such recognition is often crucial in creating a space for "something other" to emerge, a "third thing," born of the analytic interaction but slightly separate from the individual participants, a discourse less contested than shared.

# 5

# "Nothing Could Be Further from the Truth": Lack and the Analyst's Attitude

*By now the reader is familiar with the central conceptual tandem that underwrites my clinical theory: lack and desire. In this chapter I dive more deeply into this seemingly abstract idea—the analyst's lacking position—and the ways in which it informs a flexible, alive, gyroscopic way of working.*

> For the listener, who listens in the snow,
> And, nothing himself, beholds
> Nothing that is not there and the nothing that is.
>
> —Wallace Stevens, "The Snowman"

Caught yet again in a debate with his girlfriend over the lack of direction in his life, Evan feels deflated. "You always shoot me down just when I feel more hopeful about things," he tells her. Evan had started working on his back taxes, something he had put off for several years.

"That's great, you getting started with your taxes," she says, "but I'm worried your hopefulness is premature. You always think that optimism will carry you through on these things; so far, it hasn't. After all, you just started working on your taxes last night."

"Well, what do you think will carry me through, then?" Evan says, feeling lost.

"It won't be optimism alone," his girlfriend replies.

Evan says to her: "Nothing scares me more than when you say that."

It is easy for me, Evan's analyst, to get caught up in his struggles—with his girlfriend, with his taxes, with other things he says he must get done but never does. I simply repeat Evan's last statement: "Nothing scares you more than when she says that."

"Right. Nothing."

To my ear he's lost in a kind of forlorn, concrete state, a hallmark of which is his inability to hear his own speech from another perspective, to hear the fullness of what he has been saying. I am reminded of similar statements Evan has made: "There's nothing stopping me." Or, "Being unhappy is certainly better than nothing." Once I said to him that he hoped I would magically transform him, give him that "special something" so he could finally and resolutely act.

His response: "Nothing could be further from the truth."

I asked him why he felt this way.

"Because ultimately I'm on my own. It's my work to do in here. I either do it or I don't. You can help me to look at things, and I want you to point things out to me. But in the end, I'm the one that has to find a job; I'm the one that has to finish my taxes. But," he says more somberly, "I feel nothing can help me. I've been alone for so long."

The questions I explore in this chapter are two: What is this "nothing" of which Evan is so afraid? And what is this "nothing" that can be of help? Lack is a source of great anxiety and, for some, trauma ("I wish nothing *were* further from the truth"). This is the lack of emptiness, deadness, the nonvital. Andre Green's (1986) Dead Mother concept is a key example of the ways in which dead relationships, dead objects, are said to haunt the traumatized subject. In such cases lack can be terrifying. Lack is also an important condition of our relative freedom from conflict and trauma ("Nothing *can* help me"). These two questions—the nothing that is a source of fear and trauma, and the nothing that is a source of help and freedom—form the outer boundaries of my remarks. I will return to these questions, and Evan, later.

## The Analyst's Lacking Position—the Backstory

Much of the psychoanalytic literature over the past twenty-five years has elaborated a certain point of view regarding the analyst's position in the analytic process. Underwritten, I believe, by Roy Schafer's concept of action (1983), analysts such as Jacobs (1986), McLaughlin (1991), Chused (1991), Renik (1993b), and Hoffman (1994) have described in compelling fashion the analyst's inevitable, real-time—and also the analyst's fallible or flawed—involvement in the analytic process. Based on the fact that analysts as well as patients are motivated by unconscious wishes and fears, the analyst cannot help being involved and acting in unintended, unexpected, and surprising ways. Grossman (1999), among others, has written from a more epistemological point of view—less about how the analyst unwittingly gets involved with patients and more about what the analyst does not know or, as Grossman has put it, what the analyst does not hear.

For some among us, this emphasis on the analyst's involvement, and more broadly on the direct therapeutic effects of the analytic atmosphere and relationship, has not been entirely welcome, because it seems to undermine the role of rational understanding (i.e., insight) in the cure. The enactment literature forces us to struggle with this issue of meaning and insight. If the analyst is a real-time participant in the analytic field, she remains, in one way or another, a real-time interpreter as well. As a profession we are preoccupied with meaning. Yet we have also known, since Freud, that insight alone—what we might call a particular kind of psychoanalytic self-awareness—is often not curative. Insight can be of no moment.[1] While the analyst may feel the burden of having to make sense of the patient, it is not at all clear that the analyst's positive giving of meaning to the patient plays the central curative role that many have claimed for it.

Just as much of the enactment literature makes explicit reference to the analyst's role in helping patients expand their self-awareness, it also demonstrates that this expansion of self-awareness is facilitated by the analyst's *misguided actions and incorrect or errant interpretive efforts*. In other words, in these cases the analyst's being "right" does not further the analytic process; rather, the analyst's being "wrong" does. This fact suggests that the variety of the analyst's interventions—within the broad structure of the analytic frame and the analyst's role (Almond 1995)—is more important than the precise semantic content of any one so-called interpretation.

Many outside the contemporary Freudian tradition in American psychoanalysis have addressed this issue of the analyst's faulty functioning as constitutive of ongoing and often productive analytic work. Analysts of the British Independent Group have repeatedly foregrounded the patient's emerging subjectivity, aliveness, and authenticity within the analytic process and deemphasized the analyst's positive giving of information and insight. For example, Winnicott, with an unerring eye for the ironic and paradoxical, explicitly argues for a kind of optimal analytic relating in which the analyst—in order to function optimally—must fall short. For Winnicott, the analyst's failing is a necessary element in a successful analytic process. In "On Transference" (1956) Winnicott writes: "The patient makes use of the analyst's failures. ... The analyst needs to be able to make use of his failures in terms of their meaning for the patient, and he must if possible account for each failure even if this means a study of the unconscious counter-transference" (388). And in "The Use of an Object" (1969) Winnicott notes: "I think

---

[1] I discuss this question in greater detail in Chapter 10.

I interpret mainly to let the patient know the limits of my understanding" (711). The analyst must tolerate missing the patient and welcome the patient's reactions and associations to the analyst-as-missing. Casement has taken the Winnicottian ethos furthest in his two important books, *Learning from the Patient* (1985) and *Learning from Our Mistakes* (2002). Casement is keenly attentive to ways in which the analyst's overvaluing her own thinking risks collapsing the analytic space and fostering compliance in the patient. Casement's overall interest is in characterizing an optimal analytic attitude. Here is a representative offering:

> If ... the analyst is genuinely open to correction, there is a quite different security available to the patient. It does not have to be that brittle security that threatens to collapse in the face of any mistake. Instead, another kind of security can be found that is much more resilient, security that comes from the patient finding that the analyst can be corrected, even by the patient. And ... the too certain analyst is also defending a brittle security against whatever might threaten it, whether from the patient or from colleagues who could disagree. (2002, 4)

In the French tradition, Faimberg (2005) has written creatively on the centrality of "listening to listening": that is, the analyst's listening to how the patient listens to the analyst's various offerings. The analyst's consciously intended meaning takes a back seat to the retroactive meaning the patient gives the analyst's words. The analyst finds out what she "meant" in the particularity of the patient's reply. Both analyst and patient are effectively *decentered* subjects in the analytic dialogue. The uncanny otherness of our own spoken words—inevitably imbued with varieties of tone and pace and force—once they are in circulation and responded to, undermines, however slightly, both participants' assumed view of themselves and what they have said.[2]

The relational and self-psychological literature is an extended meditation on both the problems and the opportunities offered by the analyst's mistakes and misunderstandings. Kohut, of course, championed the importance of the inevitable failures of empathy on the part of the analyst. Arnold Goldberg (2004) puts misunderstanding at the very center of an effective analytic process. As I alluded to briefly in Chapter 4, Jessica Benjamin, in her paper "Beyond Doer and Done-To" (2004), writes of the analyst's recapturing

---

[2] Faimberg's (2005) rendering of an alive dialectical analytic process is a compelling view of the analytic speech relation about which I wrote in Chapter 2. Faimberg, I would say, fully "gets it."

her desire and functioning as an analyst after being caught in resistance, necessarily cocreated by analyst and patient:

> The analyst has to change ... and in many cases this is what first leads the patient to believe that change is possible. While there is no recipe for this change, I suggest that the idea of surrendering rather than submitting is a way of evoking and sanctioning this process of letting go of our determination to make our reality operative. To do this ... is to find a different way to regulate ourselves, one in which we accept loss, failure, mistakes, our own vulnerability. (32)

In another now-classic paper, Stephen Cooper (2004) describes the importance for the patient of the analyst's functioning, in part, as a "new bad object" to facilitate the inevitable emergence of the negative transference and, ultimately, new self-experience and psychological growth.

While many have offered—from seemingly quite different theoretical orientations—helpful descriptions of the importance of the analyst's mistakes to clinical process, no conceptual understanding of this point has been offered to explain it. In my estimation we don't have a good theory for why the analyst's missing the patient is not only an inevitable ingredient but also an essential one, in the natural unfolding of a successful analytic process. I argue that *nothing*, or *lack*, is central to our understanding of this ingredient. As I have noted, many have written on the clinical value of the analyst's being wrong or misguided—whether by virtue of an "incorrect" interpretation, a tactless remark, an over-hesitant offering, emotional withdrawal, or rote ways of behaving and interpreting. My hope here is to offer, in part, a theoretical basis for the oft-repeated clinical observation that missing the patient, getting it wrong, can be analytically helpful, the very basis of moving the process forward. What I will show is that the analyst, as a subject of desire, can only offer the partial, the half-said—there is always something lacking at the level of the statement or of the action, because there is something missing at the level of being.

My basic assertion is this: The analyst's missing the patient, on a fundamental level, is an evocation of lack. This missing, if tolerated by both analyst and patient, allows the patient to take up his own place, to articulate in increasingly clear ways a position in his own individual voice. As Ogden (2000) writes in "The Dialectically Constituted/Decentered Subject of Psychoanalysis," "The subject of psychoanalysis takes shape in the interpretive space *between* analyst and analysand" (224, my emphasis). The space of which Ogden writes is born of this lack, or difference, that marks each subject as subject and each and every intersubjective experience. If the psychoanalyst is a curator of space, it is her lacking position that allows for this space to open.

Although this may all sound quite abstract, in truth, I am entering this discussion from a distinctly clinical vantage point—the interesting and perplexing phenomenon of missing the patient. But I would be misleading the reader if my purview were understood as only about these moments of missing. What I am pointing toward and will attempt to explain in detail is how the concept of lack—not the concept, actually, but lack itself—what some have called the gap—is an essential element of the analyst's *basic working conditions*. These conditions include the interacting subjectivities of analyst and analysand. They also include the nature of meaning, how words and thoughts attach themselves to objects, both internal and external. In other words, the analyst's capacity not only to tolerate but inhabit a lacking position as a key feature of the analyst's desire allows the analyst's being wrong to really count as being wrong. It also allows the analyst to be right, if the patient feels the analyst says something on the mark. The point remains, however, that even if the analyst is "right," she is right *only as far as it goes*. There is always a limit or a void in any statement, even if the statement suggests an excess of meanings. If both parties in the analytic endeavor can explore this inevitable missing-in-meaning—within the interpretive space this missing creates—then the analytic process can be meaningfully furthered. The role of lack in the analytic process also suggests an additional way to conceptualize termination—this is the point at which the patient's desire for knowledge abates. Part of the interpretive attitude we hope to instill in our patients is to know when to stop interpreting. This is especially true for people with an obsessional character structure.[3]

If the analyst recognizes and tolerates this condition of lacking, it becomes a working principle of the analyst's attitude. But "working principle" makes things sound nearly juridical. Instead, I am trying here to capture something that is more like an *internal gyroscope* that is always there, ever present, though the analyst will inevitably lose contact with this "instrument" in moments of anxiety, confusion, or duress.

The analyst's constitutively lacking state, as an internal gyroscope, orients the analyst in an anticipatory, futural direction poised to engage with whatever unfolds in the now-and-the-next of the work. If the analyst is too invested in her positive presence, her "goodness," her beneficence and desire to help—the details of overvaluing presence can take myriad forms—then the natural pivoting and constant reorienting of this analytic

---

[3] In Chapter 10, I will wonder about this goal and if it is at all possible, as I consider the question of desire and the interminable nature of psychoanalytic work.

gyroscope will be constrained as the analyst, fearing the patient, fights for certain positions, and clings to a specific way of being or view of herself. I am gesturing here toward the *proleptic unconscious*, a domain I discuss in detail in Chapter 9.

As the reader can sense, I conceptualize the clinical point that missing the patient facilitates a salutary analytic process as part of a struggle the analyst (and the patient) has in dealing with his or her own lack. The analyst's struggle is in part the obsessional's struggle. Both analyst and patient are lured by the promise of understanding and closure—the hope that "figuring out what is going on" will not only lessen emotional pain but will also rid the patient, as Freud said, of "common unhappiness."

In what follows, I want to build a case for why lack is an essential working condition for both analyst and analysand. First, I discuss the role of lack in the development of systems of meaning and in the development of the human subject. Lack is constitutive both of ways of understanding (i.e., the ways we graft understanding onto the Real), and of the emergence of human subjectivity. In the following section, I grapple with the complexities within psychoanalytic theory of the object relation, and biases within our theory toward presence and plenitude (biases that serve to obscure the role of lack). Through a comparison of Klein's and Lacan's rendering of the nature of the object in the object relation, I hope to capture some of this complexity. Later in the chapter I will return to the case of Evan with this intent in mind: to show how both Evan and I struggled to deal with lack and how each of us offered up easy solutions that were obsessional in nature. Finally, I discuss in more detail the clinical implications of lack as an essential working condition of the analyst and the benefits to the analyst of embracing this condition.

For now I want to turn to a theoretical discussion of the role of lack in the development of systems of meaning and in the nature of human subjectivity.

## Meaning and the Subject: The Role of Lack

In a well-known footnote in *The Interpretation of Dreams* (1900), Freud is in the process of analyzing his Dream of Irma's Injection: "I had a feeling that the interpretation of this part of the dream was not carried far enough to make it possible to follow the whole of its concealed meaning. ... There is at least one spot in every dream at which it is unplumbable—a navel, as it were, that is its point of contact with the unknown" (111 n. 1).

Freud is working with a model of dream interpretation that posits a web of concealed meanings (the unconscious dream thoughts fueled by a wish) within or behind the manifest content of the dream. As Freud at first implies, if he had only gone further with his associations it would have been possible to follow the "whole of [the dream's] concealed meaning." But the whole of the dream is also the hole in the dream, as Freud then posits the existence of a lack in the system of meaning—that is, the dream's navel. The dialectic of meaning and its lack is fully at play in this brief but significant footnote. Here one feels Freud's passion, his intense desire to find more meaning, his satisfaction in finding it, and, simultaneously, his knowing that any understanding is necessarily incomplete. This incompleteness causes a desire for something more, a further searching and elaboration of meaning. This play of meaning's presence and the absences that necessarily haunt it is a hallmark of our work.

Andre Green (1973), in a review of Bion's *Attention and Interpretation*, emphasizes the dependence of thought's emergence on a structural limit: "At one point or another, any preconception can be subjected to the impossibility of finding its realization. The development of thought depends on this nonrealization" (117). The baby is endowed with an a priori expectation of the breast as a source for nourishment; its frustration in the face of no-breast promotes the beginnings of thought. Note here that for Bion realization or nonrealization means "reality"—what reality presents for the subject. Opatow (1997) makes a similar point regarding the psychoanalytic basis of cognition: "Cognition properly (that is, symbolically) begins when th[e] pain of instinctual need becomes experienced as lack, a negation that constitutes the wish—an awareness that something could be absent. Conceptual negation is what the mind does with instinctual pain" (883–4). From a different intellectual tradition, Searle (2001) writes that the "gap" is the basis of rational and irrational decision-making. The gap is precisely that place where choice (read: desire) is possible. Searle writes, sounding strangely Lacanian, "What fills the gap? Nothing. Nothing fills the gap: you make up your mind to do something, or you just haul off and do what you are going to do, or you carry out the decision you previously made, or you keep going, or fail to keep going in the project you have undertaken" (17). Each of these writers insists that thinking and desiring rest squarely on an experience of missing or lacking something. And, of equal importance, to claim to understand is an implicit appeal that words and thoughts cover the lack that engenders them. But the symbolic is never seamless; there is always a stain as a mark of the lack in any symbolic system. The only reason there is cause for translation, or negotiation, or giving an account is that there is something missing or awry in a given system.[4]

---

[4] In this context, it is easy to see how Laplanche's important concept of the "enigmatic message" derives from these preceding ideas about lack, desire, and what is inevitably incomplete in any utterance.

As I have suggested earlier in this chapter, lack also informs the coming into being of the human subject. Freud founded the emergence of the psychoanalytic subject on the experience of loss. Green notes as much in *The Work of the Negative* (1993): "By emphasizing the effects of lack, psychoanalytic theory was linked to the negative from the outset. If one thinks of the basic model of the mind, i.e., hallucinatory wish fulfillment, one possesses the most decisive argument for the existence of a work based on an unsatisfied wish" (56).

Lacan also emphasized desire's dependence on the lost object. Using Freud's story of the *Fort! Da!* game as a model, Lacan asserted that the child becomes a desiring subject through speaking the loss it is experiencing. The child's mother is gone; she desires elsewhere. The child speaks his desire for her. Lack and its representation occur simultaneously, each constituting the other. The well-known Lacanian statement on this point is: "the symbol first manifests itself as the killing of the thing, and this death results in the endless perpetuation of the subject's desire" ([1953] 2002, 262). Hoagy Carmichael captures the same idea in a line from the beginning of "Stardust": "You wander down the lane and far away, leaving me a song that will not die."

Lacan calls this acculturation of the child—this speaking and fantasying instead of simply being an object for the mother—symbolic castration. We give up the increasingly onerous and burdensome status as singular object of the mother's interest—her "phallic object"—in order to come into being as a desiring subject in our own right. The lack or gap that engenders desire (cognition for Opatow; choice for Searle) simultaneously gives rise to speech. To become a speaking being means, ontologically, that the unmediated object (the mother, psychoanalytically considered) must be sacrificed. The Real now becomes mediated by the Symbolic. Thus Lacan moves the issue of castration away from the specular reality of what one can see to what one must lose in order to become a subject, whether one is biologically male or female. The phallus, no longer a thing in the Real, now becomes a signifier (of power, strength, prestige, and the like), and a signifier with which both men and women can identify. We are all, then, castrated on a Symbolic level.

There is a substantial psychoanalytic literature on the importance of lack and negation in the development of the human subject that supports the theoretical point of view I am offering here. I will mention only a few key contributions. Litowitz (1999) delineates a developmental line for negation, and stresses the crucial importance of negation for the emergence of subjectivity. Fonagy and Target (1998) describe an optimal interaction between mother and child that promotes the child's inner mental experience. They caution that if the object is too present, the gap is covered over, and lack loses its generative representational possibilities: "If the [mother's] mirroring is too accurate, the perception itself can become a source of fear [for the child], and it loses its symbolic potential" (94). In such a situation the mother's presence cannot be escaped; for the child there is no choice, no possible mediation, and nothing about which to reflect. Ogden (2000) describes the emergence of subjectivity as a series of dialectical challenges. In Ogden's hands the subject struggles with certain unresolvable binary oppositions: presence/absence, conscious/ unconscious, splitting/integration, inside/outside, destruction/ reparation. Benjamin (2000) offers a similar description. She stresses the dual importance of the subject's capacity to recognize the other and also to negate it in order to achieve separation. Note that the terms in each of these signifying pairs (e.g., inside/outside, conscious/unconscious, recognition/negation) are meaningful only diacritically in relation to its opposing term. Lack resides in the space or barrier between the paired terms, allowing difference to be maintained and preventing the terms from collapsing into each other.

The foregoing can be summarized as follows: *The structure of the subject and the structure of meaning both rest on a space created by lack.*

## The Lure of Plenitude

The obsessional's question is everyone's question: How do I deal with the lack in the other and in myself? This is the flip side of the question: How do I deal with desire—always somewhat opaque—in the other and myself? The obsessional has a particular answer to these questions: to fill up the lack in the other with thinking; to imagine one knows the other's experience without listening to the other; and to misrecognize one's own ideas and experiences as the other's ideas and experiences. This is what I call the *lure of plenitude*: We have gifts to give to our patients, such as our positive presence; our knowledge, insight, and wisdom; and our emotional sensitivity. The analyst's wanting to be and to offer these "things" is, of course, caused by lack and the belief or fantasy that it can be filled. For the analyst, this appeal is not without value; it allows us to have our own personal touchstones that help us feel safer as we do our work. These touchstones are often admixtures of clinical theory, commonsense folk psychology, and identifications with colleagues, supervisors, or one's analyst. These touchstones allow us to have, at least some of the time, a "mind of one's own" (Caper 1997).

Like Shel Silverstein's Missing Piece looking for the Big O to complete it (only to stop the missing piece from exploring and seeking further), so we analysts inevitably seek sense-making tools to help us deal with the lack that marks our subjectivity and our own sense-making efforts. The concepts we use to fill this lack are what Lacan called "signifiers of the lack in the Other."

The Other, as defined by Lacan, is that which is both outside and prior to the subject's coming into being—outside in relation to the subject's conscious awareness and prior in the sense that defining institutions—language, family constellation, culture, law—predate the actual birth of the person. As Evans (1996) explains, "The big Other designates radical alterity ... [which] Lacan equates ... with language and the law, and hence the big Other is inscribed in the order of the symbolic. Indeed, the big Other is the symbolic insofar as it is particularized for each subject" (133). Inevitably, the big Other is not seamless because there is always a lack—something missing at the heart of any symbolic system. Here Laplanche's concept of the *enigmatic signifier* helps in grasping this constitutive lack, if we consider the simple fact that the child experiences his or her adult caretakers as opaque no matter how reliably empathic and available they may be; and for the child relations among adults (from mere acquaintanceship to being lovers) only come into clear view gradually, over many years, and that clarity is shot through with fantasy and desire. It is never complete.

In this sense, there can only be a series of translations (again, following Laplanche)—substitutions, stand-ins, words, and imaginings—for this lack in the Other. And yet, as a basic matter of fact one finds biases in psychoanalytic theory toward presence and plenitude. Presence is privileged and lack obscured. Everything means something; there are no gaps or lacks in the Other or in ourselves. As Reed (2002) writes in her review of Green's *The Work of the Negative*, "For Freud and the ego psychologists ... the psychoanalyst moves in a positive world in which meaning always exists to be uncovered. For Melanie Klein, too, meaning always exists. ... Both Freud and Klein think in a universe of presences, there to be interpreted" (344). In a world of positive presences (hidden or manifest), the analyst's role is to see what is there and find ways to point these observations out to the patient. The analyst's lack—the very basis of the analyst's desire—is obscured. I would call this an obsessional bias, or the analyst's obsessional discourse. When caught in the grips of this bias, the analyst's internal gyroscope stops spinning, stops moving, stops adjusting to what is before her in the clinical moment.

Among the psychoanalytic ideas that emphasize presence (and so obscure the effects of lack) is one that has had great influence in psychoanalysis and, in spite of its long history, retains great contemporary influence. This is the view that the essence of psychoanalytic practice is based on the object relation. In this view, psychoanalysis is fundamentally dyadic in nature and rests on the mother-child (or breast-infant) template. The object is not lost; the object's presence is problematic in some way for the patient, and so is, variously, defended against. This is defensive work born of a desire that "nothing could be further from the truth."

Certainly, both ego psychological (Anna Freudian) and British Independent analysts emphasize the importance of the qualities of the analyst's presence, including the analyst's attending to questions of tact and timing, levels of anxiety and the defensive structure in the patient, and the like. Bion, of course, put the mother/analyst front and center with his theory of container/contained. While it seems patently true that all psychoanalysts view analysis as based on the object relation—though the accents and stresses may be quite different—it is fair to recognize Melanie Klein's priority in this regard. It is also true that the contemporary Kleinians have seen this emphasis through to its logical clinical conclusions. I have in mind Joseph's (1989) emphasis on the "total situation" of the transference and all the technical precepts that follow from that emphasis.

Andre Green (1993) has taken some key notions from Bion, and to some extent from Klein, and brought them together with his interest in what he called the *work of the negative*. The object relation and the work of the negative are intimately related. A general description of this work of the negative in the clinical setting is that it is the work of objectification. The patient has trouble with the analyst's presence, with what the analyst has to offer: her careful listening, her interpreting, and, at least implicitly, her way of thinking. The patient also struggles with aspects of the psychoanalytic setting, such as the requirement to "say what comes to mind" (the fundamental rule). A more Kleinian emphasis pictures a patient who nullifies the analyst as an autonomous, desiring subject through splitting, projective identification, and omnipotent control of the object. The patient, in other words, attempts to collapse the analytic space and the differences and otherness the space both supports and suggests. Green's emphasis is somewhat different: the patient is seen as "phobic" about his own mind and where it might go if given free reign; in such cases, free association ceases and, instead, silence and absence are cathected. Whatever the specifics—whether one follows Green or Klein or Bion—as a general matter it can appear that the goal of a psychoanalysis based on the object relation is a gradual rectification of a dyadic—mother/infant—relationship gone awry. The analyst/maternal object is fundamentally always there, whether the patient lies on a couch or sits *vis-à-vis*; the patient defends against recognizing and dealing psychologically with this fact.

## A Clinical Critique of the Lure of Plenitude

I have asserted that much of our theory biases us in the direction of presence and plenitude. This bias, in turn, underwrites a "negative" reading of the negative, a reading that emphasizes what the patient is doing to or with the setting, and doing to the analyst. Here's the fundamental issue from my point of view: if the analyst's position is conceptualized as a positive presence—modeled on the nourishing breast and containing mother with the assumption that the analyst's interventions are essentially a "good feed"—then the analyst's role in creating resistances and impasses will not only remain hidden but will also be misrecognized as simply more benign help against which the patient defends. In this view, it is the patient who is solely responsible for the collapse of analytic space and the objectification of the other on which this collapse depends. How can the analyst take responsibility for her activity if this activity is not seen for what it is? This can be one of the costs—one that cannot be minimized—of the analyst's overemphasis on presence and plenitude.

An example of bias toward the analyst's positive presence and the patient's defense against it can be seen in an exchange between Busch and Joseph published in the *International Journal of Psychoanalysis* in 2004. Their texts are both pithy and rich, and engage several important clinical issues, the most important of which is that classic psychoanalytic debate between the proper object of analytic focus: surface versus depth. That is, ought the analyst to focus attention on that which the patient can, with a little help from the analyst, attend to and think about (Busch's view), or should the analyst address the most "primitive" anxieties and phantasies (Joseph's view)? (We will set aside the entire problematic of surface and depth, or the primitive, for that matter.) In her rejoinder to Busch, Joseph presents a dream of a female patient in her mid-twenties. In the dream the patient is in "a large place" and something goes wrong: "She was on one side of the place," Joseph tells us, "the analyst on the other. I, the analyst, took it on myself to phone for help; my patient felt resigned and sad. She queried to herself would the phone call be helpful or make more trouble since the police might burst in" (574). Joseph interprets the dream as follows:

> There is an awareness that she needs help yet the analyst is kept at great distance—in the dream at the other side of the place; in the session by the long pauses and constant withdrawal of contact that I have described. ... [The patient] splits off her need for help and the active part that could seek help, and this ... is projected into the analyst. (574)

From Joseph's point of view, the patient, because of her own anxieties about her dependency and need for help, must keep great distance from the analyst.

Busch offers a symmetrical reading of the dream:

> The dream also tells us that something goes wrong, and it is my understanding that the patient is saying this has to do with the communication from the analyst to the patient. Far away from her

patient, Joseph talks to someone else on the phone, not to the patient's conscious or preconscious ego on the other side of this place. (575)

Joseph sees the dream from the analyst's point of view and judges the patient to be defensive; Busch reads the material from the patient's viewpoint and judges the analyst to be defensive.

The question of who is right in this controversy is the wrong question. There is in fact no way of adjudicating this dispute, because the readings of the dream are symmetrical; they mirror each other. The controversy demonstrates the logical reversibility (and inherent undecidability) of the dual-relation resistance. More importantly, the controversy exposes the danger of overemphasizing the analyst's positive presence, because analysts so disposed may misrecognize their role in the interaction and not hear what the patient is trying, perhaps anxiously, perhaps haltingly, to say. The analyst who inhabits the position of lack is better able to "roll with"—gyroscope-like—that tension born of and in between the poles of presence and absence. A bias toward presence obscures the basic structure of these intersubjectively constituted and quite common resistances. The analytic space often collapses under the weight of this bias.

## The Nature of the Object-Relation

The difficulty in maintaining the analytic space is certainly more complex than I have rendered it thus far. The crucial question is how one conceptualizes the nature of the object found in the "object relation." Is the object seen as a full presence, or is the object a more complicated figure, marked by lack and desire, a presence made of a fundamental and constitutive absence? I have suggested there is a significant cost to overemphasizing the positive presence of the analyst (what amounts to— as I have just said—a particular kind of rendering of the object relation). I have also suggested, but have yet to fully spell out, the salutary benefits of biasing oneself toward lack. But excessively rigid adherence to the position of lack can lead to clinical problems similar to those one finds with a bias toward the analyst's positive presence. A comparison of Klein and Lacan demonstrates this point and shows that analysts of very different theoretical perspectives can end up privileging two sides of the same coin. Klein emphasized the analyst's presence; Lacan the analyst's absence. More broadly, Klein spoke of the object's presence; Lacan stressed the object's fundamental absence, the fact that the primary psychoanalytic object is lost.[5]

---

[5] This is a debate, in part, about the representability, or lack thereof, of the maternal object.

It is an open question which analyst tended toward plenitude. It seems reasonable to point to Klein in this regard, since the importance of the object is emphasized so strongly and lack is not theorized as such. In this tradition, the transference is taken as real and central and must be addressed by the analyst. For Lacan (1981), the transference is a lure (a kind of lack) that causes the analysand to keep talking, but an explicit focus on the transference is simultaneously a "closing up" of the unconscious, not its revelation. The analyst's commenting, for example, about the "feeling in the room," or aspects of matricial space and the frame that come up intrusively in the form of whatever has been and is happening—quite usual fare in contemporary clinical practice—such interventions are simply relegated to a failure of analytic discipline, as the analyst is said to be speaking to the patient's "ego" (rather than the "subject of the unconscious"). In other words, rigid adherence to the Lacanian view may lead the analyst to keep an unnecessary distance from the patient, and create an atmosphere in which certain things are simply not discussed and untoward feelings are tossed aside as so much "misrecognition." The risk is a deadening of the relationship. Purcell (2004) describes this deadening as an example of "attenuated countertransference" based on the analyst's theory. Far from allowing the patient maximal expressive freedom, overvaluing the analyst as absent object can create its own pressures on the patient. One can believe one is avoiding the obsessional solution by biasing oneself toward lack, but if reified and rigidly adhered to, this approach is itself an obsessional solution. Nancy and Lacoue-Labar (1992) have called Lacan's theory of the subject a "negative theology." It can become so if analysts are unable to keep a certain distance from their ideas and beliefs. Jonathan Dunn's (1995) wise counsel is relevant to this discussion: analysts must not only continually struggle to "decathect" themselves narcissistically when listening to patients, but must also constantly strive to do the same from their cherished theories as well.

Given the discussion above, a more complete description of the nature of the object in the object relation can be offered: *the object is present but necessarily lacking*. And so, *the psychoanalyst is present but necessarily lacking*. This is not merely a question of bias; it is a question of fact.

## Evan Again

The analyst has a tendency to struggle with the very concerns that plague those subjects who tend toward obsessional "solutions." These struggles inform the analyst's attitude.

As a way to further unpack the nature of these ways of dealing with lack, I want to return to Evan for a closer look. Though I have emphasized the positive or facilitative aspects of lack in the emergence of the subject, the case of Evan suggests that there are negative and deeply traumatic effects of lack as well. These effects are usually thought of as preoedipal trauma. Since my main focus is on the role of lack in the analyst's position and attitude, I will not discuss in any detail the traumatic effects of early lack and deprivation here.

Single and in his early thirties, Evan came to me some years ago at the behest of his new girlfriend, who was shocked to see how stuck he was in his life. She was also shocked that he didn't seem to be aware of it. Evan was unemployed and slowly depleting the small amount of savings he had received from his parents. He told himself he would, at any moment, return to school to complete his BA. He had only two classes to go. Yet for the past six years he had not picked up the application for readmission. His father was a successful businessman and philanthropist. Because of Evan's procrastinating ways, however, his parents had ceased to help him financially with the exception of paying, in part, for his treatment.

The oldest of five children, Evan struggled with anger and loneliness throughout much of his childhood. His parents were dutiful but distant. Of particular relevance is that his mother nearly died in giving birth to him and was medically compromised during the first weeks of his life. She eventually recovered. Evan felt alone with feelings he didn't understand. Though bright and capable, as a teenager he dropped out of high school, bummed around and did odd jobs. He was briefly married, and eventually he got his high school equivalency degree. Though admitted to university after two years at a junior college, he had yet to graduate, six years later.

Early on in the analysis, Evan felt everything to be impossible. He often arrived at my office bearing the burden of a huge weariness. He lay down and sighed. He often cried. One would have thought he was gearing up to climb Mount Everest. Instead he was feeling the weight of going to the grocery store or the bank. He spoke in a dreamy way, in order to stay calm. He fell into self-justification and cheerleading whenever he decided to do something, even a task like the ones just mentioned. To decide was to die, so intensely did he want to hold on to all possibility. He set up conditions utterly irrelevant to the decision at hand in order to make it or, more usually, to not make it. Evan not only felt decisions to be impossible—he identified with impossibility itself.

Yet Evan kept searching for answers. He implored his parents to tell him why they had been so passive all these years: "How did you understand what I was going through? Couldn't you see how unhappy I was? Did you ever think to ask? Jesus fucking Christ!"

These are important questions, and, if put forward with less insistence and demand, could be possible avenues of communication and understanding. But Evan was trying to extract something from his parents: an answer so indelible, so rock-solid, that it would never go away. This effort, too, staged an impossibility, because no question is answerable in the totalizing way Evan demanded. Like all speech that attempts to describe—forever marking a trail to the truth rather than leading to a final destination—no answer can be complete and, therefore, no answer entirely adequate. Evan had a fantasy that there were such answers. He had succumbed to the lure of plenitude. Once his father or mother produced the answer that was definitive, no other questions would need to be asked. Then, finally, Evan could move forward. But there were no such answers. Evan was stuck.

Evan was anxious and unmoored about this lack in the other. At times I was as well. Often I would say something quite straightforward to him. Just as often he would ask me to say it again, which I would do. After a while, as this pattern continued, I stopped repeating what I had said. Evan's response was varied but always troubled. He said he couldn't remember my exact words and it felt really important that he remember them. But in a more subtle way he needed to fix my words so they remained mine—frozen in time—while he stayed unmoved and untouched. When he would request a repeat interpretation, I would say nothing, or ask him what he remembered, or inquire why he was asking or what was getting in the way of his remembering. But the most difficult thing to say to him was "I don't know exactly what I meant," or "I don't exactly remember," or "You want time to stand still and my words not to count." Earlier in the analysis my lack of understanding or uncertainty about something often caused him deep despair. Obviously, I tried to stay interested in how he felt I had missed him.

My alluding to the possible effects of early maternal deprivation—"I think we are in territory you can't remember but that likely had a profound effect on this intense feeling of emptiness"—tended to fall flat. "I just can't remember that," Evan would say. "We're living it," I would reply. "Maybe," he would say.

Evan was better able to elaborate the nature of his present despair. He felt, he said, "up against it." He was scared to feel overt disappointment or anger toward me. He told me that that felt too dangerous. He needed me too much. Yet he missed sessions and had dreams that things were falling apart.

Evan seemed to stage this lack in the Other to revisit, yet again, the point of absence and disappointment, and in this way never really to move on. I will mention a few examples. He did, eventually, get a full-time job. This was a big step for him. But uneasy about unfinished business, when home at night after work, he distracted himself. He was drawn to the television and channel-surfed. He'd skip from one show to another, feeling antsy and uncomfortable. "No, that's not it," he said to himself. "Let's find something else. No, that's not it either." Something similar happened when he attended a social event, like a party. He always felt there may be a "more happening" party somewhere else. Yet if he left one party for another, he found the next one lacking in the same way. Finally, during the first few years of analysis, he asked his parents for "help." He was not sure what such help would consist of; he just wanted it. But whatever his parents suggested (whom he might call about a possible job, for example) felt insufficient. This bothered him tremendously. When in this state of mind, in which his omnipotence was repeatedly thwarted, he wished that nothing could be further from the truth.

As the analysis progressed, there were other times, which became more frequent, when Evan would catch a glimpse of the other side, the place of a certain freedom from the obsessional search for the fully sufficient answer. This is the place where "nothing can help me." How he got his full-time job as a paralegal is an example. He had been working at a local law firm part-time, and he was well-liked. The full-time offer that came his way caused him great consternation. He worried and obsessed, and imagined all sorts of impossibilities. How, for example, would he ever make his appointments with me if he were working full-time? He pondered the pluses and minuses of the offer from every angle. But one session, in the midst of this ruminating, he stopped himself: "Here I am again wanting there to be the clearest possible path for me to take, so I don't have to make a choice. There's no way I can know in advance how this will turn out, yet somewhere I must believe I can know such things. There may be no right and wrong answers, just different ones." Then, after a pause, he struck a more somber tone: "I don't want to believe decisions can be made easily, that somehow all of this is easy, or at least not as hard as I make it. Then how would I account for the past few years where I've walked around half-dead?"

Around the time Evan took the full-time job he reported the following experience after arriving at my office on a fine spring morning: "I was riding my bike through your neighborhood. It's lovely outside. And for the first time I noticed the houses around here. Really noticed them. As I rolled by I looked at one and then another. They all looked beautiful and I felt—it was a new feeling—that I really wanted to own a house." Given Evan's propensity for pseudo-optimism, and that the day before he had been expressing his usual despair, I asked him if he was somehow propping himself up with dreams of home ownership to deal with his despairing feelings. He replied with an impressive forthrightness: "No, I don't think so. I know I do do that. But who's being repetitive now, Doc?" He chided me for what seemed to him to be a rote interpretation, at once elevating and debunking me by calling me "Doc." "No, this is different. What I'm telling you is that I felt alive as I was coming here. I was actually awake. It's so unusual for me to feel I want something."

In these two examples Evan shows signs of grappling with the "nothing" that at other times frightens him so much. With the job offer, he senses strongly enough that there is no way he can sample the future to know if a given decision is the "right" decision. In the other instance he tolerates my rather clumsy defense interpretation and is able to make clearer the rare and different feeling he had been trying to convey to me. Such an intervention could have led to his feeling put down or thinking that I was threatened by his desire—typical outcomes with interventions that are obsessional in tone or content. Instead there was a sense of playfulness in his chiding me for resorting to one of my more rote interventions in the midst of his trying to tell me that he was experiencing something new. He let me know about my own repetitiveness and my need for it.

Later in our work, Evan did return to university and finish his degree, but not without difficulty as procrastination continued to haunt him. After quite a while of hesitations and fitful starts, I suggested that he bring his computer into sessions with me to work on his final paper. He agreed. Often he worked in silence. There was the occasional, "How does this sound to you?" Eventually Evan completed his paper and graduated.

## Analytic Attitude and Lack

Why do we (both our patients and ourselves) wish that nothing could be further from the truth? Because to recognize and confront how one puts together one's place in the world—that is, sees the fantasmatic nature of one's fantasies—is upsetting, uncomfortable, and at times terrifying. Bion (1970) writes of walking in "fear and dread" (46); Lacan speaks of "subjective destitution," which "occurs when something in the fantasy wavers and makes the components of the fantasy appear" (22). When the components of the fantasy appear, the lack that supports and is hidden by the fantasy can be "seen," or experienced. This experience is the experience of nothing, and more precisely that nothing which supports what one thinks, where one is, and what one feels. It is an experience of confusion, of utter not knowing. One can see then what one has used, psychically, to prop oneself up, so to speak. What I am getting at here is not unlike that moment I described in Chapter 2 in the case of Joan: the sense that things could fall apart in an instant, since the Symbolic order is held together by unconscious assumption and implicit agreement, not physical bonds.

It is potentially quite a task for the analyst to maintain an availability to her lacking position. It takes, as Bion has emphasized, faith and passion. It takes, in other words, a particular kind of analytic desire. If we believe lack is an essential condition for the emergence of subjectivity—for the basis of mediation and self-representation—it likewise must be an essential aspect of the analyst's consciously held attitude. For the analyst, such an attitude has several advantages. First, we place implicit trust in the analytic process and in the patient with whom we are engaged. We are less invested in our own particular position and narcissistic concerns, and more committed to attending and listening to how the patient speaks, to what he says and doesn't say. How, further, he listens to himself and, following Faimberg, how he listens to the analyst. In this view of clinical process, the interpretive burden falls more equally on the patient and analyst. This promotes the patient's autonomy, his thinking, and communicates a belief to the patient that transformation is possible. Lack also encourages the analyst to consider the nature of her desire as it is impacting the patient in the now-and-the-next of the work. Obviously, the analyst must be involved with the patient in ways her understanding only partially grasps. On a related point, it is not only "okay" not to know; it is also crucial to grasp the salutary limits of the analyst's knowledge. The analyst is a curator of space. She offers what she feels and thinks, always in the service of furthering the analytic dialogue in the pursuit of truth, a pursuit that is ever-evolving but whose object is consistently in focus.

These advantages are the product of a specific, consciously held bias. Biases are inevitable in analysis. I am advocating a bias that acknowledges the lack inherent in desire, meaning, and subjectivity—a bias, in other words, that takes full account of symbolic castration. The terrain opened up by this habitation of lack is precious, as human living and expression "live" exactly there, and nowhere else.

In Chapter 6 I offer a more detailed comparison of Bion and Lacan—regarding the analyst's position and the role of desire, speech, and understanding within a psychoanalytic treatment.

# 6

## The Analyst as Listening-Accompanist: Desire in Bion and Lacan

*I wrote in Chapter 2 that the analyst is an innkeeper whose central task, in addition to the comfort and care of her charge, is to inquire about, listen to, and respond to her visitor's story. What is the innkeeper's position as she bends her ear to the wayfarer's tune? She is, in essence, her visitor's interlocutor, arguably an interlocutor of the most exquisite kind. Here I consider Bion and Lacan, two key figures in psychoanalysis, through the lens of this fundamental clinical question: what is the nature of the analyst's desire as she engages in this most unusual work of psychoanalysis? My answer is that the analyst is a listening-accompanist.*

*A space must be maintained or desire ends.*

—Anne Carson, *Eros the Bittersweet*

As I've labored to convey throughout this book, the locus of desire in psychoanalytic thought has, historically, been sought almost exclusively within the patient—his demands, transference fantasies, urgent requests, and more subtle pressures exerted in the analyst's direction. As a category of the *analyst's* experience and conceptualization, desire has been—variously—of uncertain, vague, or in some quarters, had nonexistent status. With the exception of Lacanianism and its offshoots, the analyst's desire as a direct object of analytic inquiry has been sadly lacking. Without desire as a category of inquiry, the analyst is at a substantial navigational loss and is often left to ponder faint glimmerings in the twilight of the countertransference without realizing that it is precisely her desire—the particular wishful form it has taken in that moment—that determines the countertransference to begin with, a topic I will discuss in detail in Chapter 7.

Unlike many other health-care disciplines in which standard practices for most illnesses are in fact accepted by the community, psychoanalysis is peculiar, if not unique, in that its practical efficacy is dependent on the desire of the practitioner as it affects the patient. While this statement may seem like a truism regarding any human endeavor, in psychoanalysis our practices and the analyst's desire that underwrites them often become, out of therapeutic necessity, an object of scrutiny for both analyst and analysand. (By contrast, an appendectomy is performed successfully without the desire of the surgeon becoming a necessary topic of discussion as part of that intervention, let alone a part of what is therapeutic about it.)

While this "practitioner's desire" may include knowing and even adhering to "standard practices," we might wonder whether the desire of the analyst that is efficacious has anything to do with practices that are "standard." By standard practices I mean those that should get established, over time, in any given psychoanalysis. Reliability, consistency, presence … these ways of being must be descriptive of any psychoanalyst; they get established anew in each and every intensive therapy or psychoanalysis. We might justifiably say that the analyst's reliability, consistency, and presence are key psychoanalytic virtues; within any given analysis, they become—again, over time—expected, relied on. As I discussed in Chapter 2, they constitute a matricial field of caretaking, a form of ethical responsibility for the other (Chetrit-Vatine 2014). Some have called these aspects of practice the analytic frame—they establish the formal shape of psychoanalytic work. The frame is inhabited, vivified, by these analytic virtues, that are, as I said, the backbones of essential practice.

Against this formal background of caretaking live the rhythms and happenings of the psychoanalytic hour: the anticipatory "pre-greeting" of the patient (which in the mind of the analyst may entail seconds to days), meeting her or him in the waiting room, and then listening, engaging, asking, and a thousand other things … as well as disruptions, hesitations, false starts. All of this unfolding is part of the un-accepted, the un-usual, the what-is-happening-now-and-next. For Bion and Lacan, as I describe in this chapter, this now and this next are where the desire of the analyst lives. It lives in the absence, the space, in which something new might emerge. Much can be brought to bear on any given clinical moment, on any given *here*—from the analyst's purely spontaneous gesture to an intervention that carries a substantial load of history or thought, for either the analyst or the analysand, or at times for both. Whether a light or heavy load is brought to bear, the fact remains that the moment of impact remains, shimmering in history or not, as it moves into the future. And this impact—small or not so small—is the direct result of the analyst's desire as a fact of the matter, no less consequential than a billiard ball set in motion causing a second, stationary ball to itself get going. Obviously, causation in mental functioning or in human interaction is complex and usually overdetermined. And we know that in psychoanalysis causality is bidirectional, both forward and backward, following the logic of *après-coup*. But the aspect of things the analyst has at least a chance to come into conversation with is her desire as it presses on the patient and on the analytic work.

To my mind, Bion and Lacan have surveyed this territory of the desire of the analyst most compellingly, though an explicit pairing of the two is rare in the literature.[1] Perhaps this is because, on a superficial level, the difference between them as regards desire appears to be stark: one says no to desire, the other says yes. And yet—perhaps surprisingly, perhaps not—they both situate the analyst in the same open, present, and *futural* position. This analytic position is mobile and gyroscopic (rather than static and fixed), and partakes of a particular kind of desire: *one that has not been reduced to a wish* but is, instead, trained on the unfolding moment, the emergence of something new or urgently present, something, that is, of potential significance that could not have been imagined or predicted but demands attention and respect. As the rock-bottom thing that motivates human action, desire is the genus within which various wishes are its species. Freud spoke of unconscious wishes that are threatening to consciousness and so are pressed back, or repressed. The desire I am speaking of here subsumes the Freudian *Wunsch*. Human desire, then, is a substantive in that it exists in reality. It is not, however, anything concrete. Wishes have specific and definable aims; desire, in the Lacanian sense, does not and so is "indestructible" (Lacan [1953] 2002, 431).

The distinction between wish and desire is a fruitful way forward in thinking through the role of desire in Bion's and Lacan's conceptualization of the analyst's position in clinical work. But this distinction is not an entirely stable one, as can be appreciated by considering the following questions— questions that all psychoanalysts must answer for themselves: What does the analyst want in this work, with this patient, at this time? What is it that the analyst moves toward as she listens? What, among all the "data" that the analyst encounters, must the analyst respect, take notice of, think about, and perhaps comment on, no matter what? What is the analyst willing to avow, to commit to, to stake a claim on, in the psychoanalytic endeavor? To risk, perhaps, hurting the patient for the larger purpose of helping him consider something hard, something difficult, or something that is impossible to do anything about? And what can the analyst ignore, or discount, or move beyond without undue concern or obsessive worrying? When must the analyst circle back and attend to something that had been passed over the first or second time around? These are some of the questions that I subsume

---

[1] Notable exceptions include Eigen ([1981] 1999) and Webb and Sells (1995).

under the category of the desire of the analyst.[2] They are questions that can be read as analytic wishes, especially if they take on the ossified character of the presumed, the taken-for-granted. There is an inevitable tendency to reduce the radical openness of desire—its nonconcreteness—to something specific, practical, and concrete. As will become clearer over the course of this chapter, desire is an ideal point, a stance to which the analyst aspires asymptotically, but one that in practice is less than pure and never fully reached. This *lack* in the center of desire's function and activity can never be closed or satisfied. That the desire of the analyst is a position that is, perhaps, more aspirational than achievable does not in any way nullify the importance of this specific aspiration, let alone the category of desire itself.

My effort in this chapter is partial and interpretive. I offer you a reading and intertextual analysis of a few key writings of Bion and Lacan (and some secondary sources) that mark the territory of the analyst's desire, its veritable longitude and latitude, which includes the field of language and speech as well as the nether reaches beyond this field: the Real, O, the unsymbolizable, lack—realms that are literally beyond the pale of representation and the Symbolic order. Bion, I argue, does not (and cannot) eschew desire entirely. His effort is to find the basic elements of the analyst's most effective position. Bion's pithy advice that the analyst ought to remain watchful of desire points the way toward an ideal analytic position in which a *particular* desire of the analyst is finely honed, shorn of specific wishes. This ideal position has distinct features, mostly involving *containing*, *reverie*, and *intuition*. This analytic position is one of desire, nonetheless. For Lacan, the intimate relevance of the analyst's desire to clinical work is not an issue. Instead, the analyst's question is always, what kind of desire? What is the "force-element," as Lacan says, that the analyst exerts or applies that makes an impactful difference for the analysand?

There are important differences between these two psychoanalytic thinkers, especially regarding the role of speech and language in psychoanalysis. For Lacan, desire emerges within speech driven by the demand for love and knowledge the patient makes on the analyst. For Bion, the relationship between language and desire is not theorized as such, and its role in psychoanalysis, therefore, is less clearly articulated than what one finds in Lacan. Consequently, the objects of psychoanalytic interest—what the desire of the analyst is trained on—are different for Bion and Lacan. Bion

---

[2] Jay Greenberg (2015) approaches these questions from a somewhat different angle, linking the analyst's theory of therapeutic process, which he calls a "controlling fiction," to the "analyst's responsibility" to attend and intervene in ways consistent with that theory. See Chapter 8 for further discussion of Greenberg's ideas.

emphasizes *intuition* and *emotional experience* that he believes lie outside language and secondary process functioning. For Lacan, intuition is a vague and untrustworthy ally in a practice that is fundamentally structured on the speech relation. Though these differences are important to chart, both Lacan and Bion (especially the later Bion, ca. 1967 and beyond) view the unconscious as emergent, the *to-be-realized*, and not ontic, substantial, real, reified.

Because the unconscious is "preontological," as Lacan would put it, I argue that for both Bion and Lacan the pursuit of the unconscious is ultimately an ethical pursuit, in that the psychoanalyst must tie her actions (and accounts for those actions) in relation to its emergence in the now-and-the-next of the clinical moment.[3] Lacan made the connection between desire, the unconscious, and ethics explicit (1981, 1992). Bion's emphasis on *negative capability*, on the analyst's *faith* and *passion*, the pursuit of *at-one-ment* and O, all suggest an ethics of analytic action, though as far as I know he never located the analyst's activity within an ethical field.

## Bion on Desire

Consider heartily Bion's advising the psychoanalyst to approach each session "without memory and desire" (1967). Bion writes:

Obey the following rules:

1. Memory: Do not remember past sessions. The greater the impulse to "remember" what has been said or done, the more the need to resist it.
2. Desires: The psychoanalyst can start by avoiding any desires for the approaching end of the session (or week, or term). Desires for results, "cure" or even understanding must not be allowed to proliferate. (Quoted in Spillius 1988, 18)

These "rules" have become shibboleths in contemporary psychoanalysis, perhaps because of what appear to be Bion's draconian pronouncements on desire's lures and dangers. In general, categorical statements lead to either their adherence or their dismissal. So, let's take a step or two back from

---

[3] As Lear writes: "The ethics of psychoanalysis is basically concerned with two questions: first, what is psychoanalysis good for? Second, how does psychoanalytic technique facilitate (or impede) that good?" (2012, 1244).

the manifest and categorical and think about what Bion is getting at here regarding the analyst's ideal position. In my reading, he means something like this: as we engage the patient before us, we aim to put aside what we think we know, what we remember to have been, what theoretical ideas impress upon us as we listen ... and, also, to eschew images of the future, from hopes we might have for our patient, from ideas of cure, and from such prosaic near-term interests as what we might have for dinner once the final session of the day is concluded. As Bion says in his Los Angeles Seminars, ca. 1967:

> I would like you to consider what is meant by the word desire. I am saying ... take a simple example, because I say, "Don't desire the end of the session." "Don't desire the weekend break." If you do, it will interfere with your observations. There is something very peculiar about desire. It has a peculiarly devastating effect upon one's clinical observation. (2013, 6)

Bion is trying to articulate a way—perhaps we might say an analytic method, though that word already approaches something too fixed—that creates a clearing of the psychoanalytic field of the detritus of what's already been, so that the analyst can be in the best position to engage or receive or initiate something other than received wisdom, the habitual, the already thought, the presumed known. This is a kind of eidetic reduction[4] known to phenomenology: a method of bracketing sense experience in the effort to expose the object of interest as it is, in this case, in Bion's idiom, *emotional experience*, what he termed O.[5] The Bionian project is the emptying of self (i.e., of "memory and desire") in order to receive and contain the emotional experience evolving in the session. Though "emotion" is a complex and heterogeneous term, Bion seems to mean a kind of unarticulated psychic pain that resists symbolization and gets passed between the analytic pair. The desire of the analyst at this point is to change the form of the emotional experience, to "transform" it. The analyst or patient may name this experience, but in so doing this naming both marks a piece of what-has-been

---

[4] From Wikipedia: "Eidetic reduction is a technique in the study of essences in phenomenology whose goal is to identify the basic components of phenomena. Eidetic reduction requires that a phenomenologist examine the essence of a mental object, be it a simple mental act, or the unity of consciousness itself, with the intention of drawing out the absolutely necessary and invariable components that make the mental object what it is. This reduction is done with the intention of removing what is perceived, and leaving only what is required."

[5] Let us note, in passing, the inevitable use of the language of desire to convey Bion's basic idea: "we aim to put aside"; "Bion is trying to articulate"; "in the effort to expose".

(i.e., something that has been traversed) and points to the futural unknown. "What is of importance," Ogden writes in a valuable paper on Bion, "when the analyst is ready to make an interpretation, is the unknown, which is alive even as the analyst is making an interpretation of what is already known" (2015, 296). This unknown—a place of absence from which something new can come into being—links Bion with Lacan.

Bion is taking an axe to desires in the plural, as in a "wish for this outcome" and a "wish for that object." He is not foreclosing desire per se. Simply put, Bion fashions a more refined, articulate, incisive, and present analytic desire, not the total abrogation of desire. This desire is Bion's attempt to put the analyst in the best possible position to contain, and perhaps interpret, the "emotional storm" that is inevitably created when "two personalities meet" (1994, 247). This "storm," as Hinze points out, is directly related to the patient's "demand," which Freud cautioned the analyst not to "influenc[e] ... by granting or refusing an illusory emotional satisfaction" (Freud 1927, as quoted in Hinze 2015, 767).

Regarding what I would call this *Bionian desire*, Bion himself would have had no complaint about naming it as such. It is unfortunate that his justly famous article on "memory and desire" has been so frequently misunderstood, and, frankly, misapplied, to the detriment of psychoanalytic work and theory-building. The casualty here is the crucial category of desire itself as it applies to the analyst, a category that has been relegated by many analysts to the dustbin of the unthought, or the "bad," or that which should be simply jettisoned. I cannot improve on this extended and directly relevant comment from Michael Shulman:

> "Without desire" in Bion's famous precept pertains to the analyst's "local" and immediate functioning within the session, in which open receptivity is privileged over other psychoanalytic values; it is not a recommendation for a lack of investment in the patient. The analyst's working "without desire" is close kin to Freud's "evenly suspended attention," and is an aspirational statement. It speaks to an *ideal* receptivity—the imaginary "asymptote" to the analyst's actual listening to his patient—rather than of the error-ridden, bumpy learning-curve process of actually coming to understand each patient. The phrase is absurd if taken literally, as are those notions of the analyst's eliminating memory and history to which it is linked in Bion. His is a commentary on openness and minimal pre-judgment, the analyst's *striving* to listen as much as he can, without an immediate agenda and with minimal therapeutic zeal. The analyst cannot eliminate desire, or memory, in an analytic process any more than he can eliminate knowing its history; he can only strive to limit their intrusion

on his conscious mental process and, to an extent that Bion makes quite clear is limited, on his preconscious receptive processes. Desire, here in the form of Bion's intention toward unprejudiced listening, cannot be eliminated from any human action. (2016, 714, italics in original)

The difficulty, in short, is that too often Bion's "aspirational statement" becomes yet another way for the analyst to mask her own activity and the desire that underwrites it, a topic I will discuss in relation to the issue of countertransference in Chapter 7.

## Lacan on Desire

In *The Four Fundamental Concepts of Psychoanalysis,* Lacan places the desire of the analyst in the forefront of clinical work and theorizes its explanatory potential, including the entire realm of the countertransference. Late in the seminar he observes wryly that it is entirely possible for someone "not to want to ejaculate" or "that someone may not wish to think" (1981, 234). Desire, he says, is of a different order and is more basic: "But what does not wanting to desire mean? The whole of analytic experience—which merely gives form to what is for each individual at the very root of his experience—shows us that not to want to desire and to desire are the same thing" (1981, 235).[6]

Lacan's point is consistent with what I averred about Bion's position earlier: desire is unavoidable. The question will always be, what kind of desire? As we saw from Bion, the analyst's desire is a highly refined desire—aspirational, as Shulman notes, ideal perhaps, asymptotic, as well as open, receptive, and leaning in an unknown futural direction. For Lacan, these features obtain, but he adds an element that the category of desire cannot help but suggest: the element of *force*. And so, a page or two later in the seminar, Lacan sets the scene of the psychoanalytic encounter, as the desire of the patient (whether shrouded in "not wanting to desire" or not) and that of the analyst come upon each other, as it were, "face to face." (Note the similarity with Bion's depiction of "two personalities meeting.") The patient wants something from the analyst—the analyst's love, let's say, or special knowledge.

---

[6] We might wonder if Lacan had Bion in mind here. They had met in 1945, when a contingent of French analysts visited London and spent a few weeks taking in the Kleinian scene. Bion made a singular impression on Lacan, who at that point was just emerging from the humiliation of the German occupation and a liberation that was only weeks old. Lacan wrote about this meeting: "The flame of creation burns within him; we are in the presence of one of those beings who are solitary in even their highest achievements" (Aguayo 2017, 98).

The analyst qua analyst wants something else. While Lacan paints a picture of inevitable and necessary conflict between the two parties, he also captures the subtle intensity of the analyst's ethical responsibility to the patient in the pursuit of the truth of his or her desire:

> It is at this point of meeting that the analyst is awaited. In so far as the analyst is supposed to know, he is also supposed to set out in search of unconscious desire. This is why I say ... that desire is the axis, the pivot, the handle, the hammer, by which is applied the force-element, the inertia, that lies behind what is formulated at first, in the discourse of the patient, as demand, namely, the transference. The axis, the common-point of this two-edged axe, is the desire of the analyst, which I designate here as an essential function. And let no one tell me that I do not name this desire, for it is precisely this point that can be articulated only in the relation of desire to desire. (1981, 235)

Notice the metaphors of force and action Lacan employs. The analyst uses a particularly effective kind of "internal leverage"[7] in the service of making or marking a difference to the patient at that moment. This basic point is central to any viable psychoanalytic practice: the analyst's desire not only must be brought to bear on the desire of the patient, she cannot help but bring it to bear on the desire of the patient.

There remains to be described in more detail, however, the analyst's role in causing, initiating, or venturing into moments of analytic significance and the various materials that are the objects of the analyst's desire. With respect to the analytic object one finds significant differences between Bion and Lacan, especially regarding the question of the role of speech and language in psychoanalytic work.

## Bion on Language

One key aspect of sense experience that Bion encouraged analysts to bracket is the realm of verbal meanings. He expressly distrusted the capacity of linguistic tools adequately to convey emotional experience as it evolved within a session. Again, here is Bion from the Los Angeles seminars:

> Over and over again, one is dealing with something which is as obvious and unarguable as anxiety, or sex. It is perfectly obvious to us as analysts

---

[7] I am indebted to Dr. Bo Houston for this most apt phrase.

who were in that analytic situation, but the moment we start putting it into words, it sounds like nonsense. And so it is, because the language that we use is talking about something quite different, and there's a gap between what the words mean and what they are accepted as meaning, and the thing that we're really talking about. The analytic situation with which we are all familiar is ineffable; it cannot be known except by the person who was there, and who went through that emotional experience. (2013, 4)

Bion's use of language—his particular style of literary production—has been oft-commented on; Webb and Sells (1995), for example, call it a form of "unsaying" (198). However, Bion himself said surprisingly little about language and speech as they relate to psychoanalysis. His notion of the "Language of Achievement" (1970, 125–9)—in which the analyst lives in the realm of not knowing and tolerates frustration sustained by "negative capability" in order to be open to other registers beyond linguistic representations—is more a suggestive description of the analyst's task than a worked-out theory of the role of language in analysis.[8] As a general matter, Bion seemed both to take language for granted regarding those patients who can make use of words to represent their experience (i.e., "neurotic" structures) and to minimize it for those who cannot (i.e., "psychotic" structures). Given Bion's enduring interest in and experience with patients on the borderline/schizophrenic spectrum, as his early papers such as "Attacks on Linking" (1959) demonstrate, it is no surprise that his view of language is classically Freudian: language (i.e., "word presentations") serves solely secondary process functions and so is associated with the workings of consciousness. "Bion," as Markman observes, "used the notion of caesura to indicate a divide between representations and the undifferentiated zone" (2015, 954). So Bion directs the analyst's attention to the unconscious, which, for him, is beyond language because more primitive (i.e., "psychotic") experience is in the realm of the unrepresented, the undifferentiated. (In contemporary thinking, this is the realm of trauma and dissociated/split off experience.) And as we've just seen, Bion expresses considerable worry about the capacity of words to represent psychoanalytic experience with any success.[9]

---

[8] Grotstein (1997) distinguishes between the "language of substitution—that is, of signs, symbols, and representations" and the Language of Achievement, "the hard-won yield of emotional truths that surface from the analyst's unconscious to his conscious awareness in reverie—as if they, not the analyst, were their agent" (72). Notice that this description may depend on language but barely theorizes its role in psychoanalytic work.

[9] Bion's point is entirely in keeping with my critique of narrative found in Chapter 3.

Bion is hardly the first Englishman to bemoan the limits of words to securely attach themselves to objects in the world. As Peters (1999) describes in his masterful *Speaking into Air: A History of the Idea of Communication*, there is "a long British tradition distrusting the deceit of words found in such thinkers as Bacon, Hobbes, Locke, Hume, Bentham, and Russell" (13).[10] By either taking language and speech for granted or minimizing their role altogether, Bion essentially performs an "end-around" language, speech, and the signifier. These are not, for Bion, the principal tools at the psychoanalyst's disposal. Instead, Bion increasingly pushes for the use of the analyst's *intuition* (2013, 38) and the free play of the analyst's imagination (which Bion termed *reverie*) directed toward emerging emotion that signifies aspects of psychic reality with which the patient (and often the analyst) is struggling in the session. He compares the analyst's receptivity of emotional experience (O) to that of the mystic's contact with God as the representative of truth (49). And this God is unknowable. For Bion, the analyst's desire is for emotional experience of a kind that cannot be captured by verbal means, experience that he likens to the "invisible aspects of the [electromagnetic] spectrum" (60).

There is something both compelling and vague about this picture of psychoanalytic engagement. The desired-for receptive state that the analyst ought to inhabit—this is clear enough. At the same time, there is the ever-elusive question of what the "actual emotional truth of the session" (Markman 2015, 953) means, in that the phrase suggests that *one* truth emerges. A further question is what the analyst is to do after that, once "emotional experience" is in fact experienced. The analyst, usually after considerable struggle, engages with it, thinks about it relatively open-mindedly, freely. This is the essence of what Bion called *alpha function*. And what might the analyst say about it? Often enough, words must, in the end, be summoned. Typically, Bion gives brief clinical examples of interventions that are denotative, "deep," internal to the patient, and seemingly specific. Ogden (2016) calls this "direct discourse" (414–17). For instance, in his Los Angeles seminars Bion describes patients who expressed a fear that "they would injure themselves" or who had a "dream in which they had actually cut their veins while having a bath." Bion continues:

---

[10] Sterne, in his *Tristram Shandy* ([1759] 1940), a text deeply influenced by Lockean ideas, writes: "Now you must understand that not one of these [explanations] was the true cause of the confusion in my uncle Toby's discourse. ... What it did arise from, I have hinted above, and a fertile source of obscurity it is,—and ever will be,—and that is the unsteady use of words which have perplexed the clearest and most exalted understandings ... 'Twas not by ideas,—by Heaven!; his life was put in jeopardy by words" (86–7).

I would have said: "You feel that you have something very bad inside you. And although you describe this as something which is outside of you and slashes your wrists and arms and so forth, actually I think it is felt to be an object which is inside you, which has no regard for your personality or even your anatomy, but breaks out by cutting you inside outwards." (2013, 62)

It is important to note an irony that is fairly loud here: language, it is asserted, is inherently wobbly and not to be trusted to capture an experience that is "ineffable"; yet Bion uses words as if they are functionally unproblematic, as if words precisely match experience.[11]

## Lacan on Language and the Speech Relation

Lacan's basic assessment of the limitations of language is no different from Bion's, but for Lacan this is only a so-called limitation. The "gap between what the words mean ... and the thing that we're really talking about," as Bion observed, is that gap that Lacan theorizes between *signifier* and *signified*. But unlike Bion, Lacan had a worked-out theory of the signifier—a sophisticated way of conceptualizing degrees of freedom between the word (signifier: its material sound or typography) and its various referents (i.e., signifieds). The subject represents herself and is represented by signifiers as a way of making sense of her position in the world (e.g., I am a "woman," a "student," "lonely," "happy," etc.). Without our diving deeply into territory that many others have described in detail,[12] the key points are the following: (1) the relationship between the sound or typography of a word (signifier) and its meaning (signified) is arbitrary and, also, not fixed; (2) signifiers refer in a systematic way to other signifiers, as the example of a dictionary entry demonstrates; and (3) the *signifier* is the carrier of desire and is emergent, a pointing toward other signifiers; the *signified* is meaning proper, static, fixed. This last point is especially important. In psychoanalysis the signifier is, as Lacan says below, the "mainspring," not of a specific signification but of emergent and futural signifying. Here Lacan is speaking to a group of analysts attending his 1955–6 seminar on the psychoses:

---

[11] In one of the few direct references to the analyst's use of language, Bion says: "If you use very few words, and if you always use them correctly—meaning relating directly to what you think or feel yourself—then the patient may gradually understand the language which is spoken by [the analyst]" (2005, 5).

[12] See, e.g., Benvenuto and Kennedy (1986), Evans (1996), and Fink (1995). See also Lacan (1993, 32, 119–20, 167).

I'm at sea, the captain of a small ship. I see things moving about in the night, in a way that gives me cause to think that there may be a sign there. How shall I react? If I'm not a human being, I shall react with all sorts of displays, as they say—modeled, motor, and emotional. I satisfy the description of psychologists, I understand something, in fact I do everything I'm telling you that you must know how not to do. If on the other hand I am a human being, I write in my log book, *"At such and such a time, at such and such a degree of latitude and longitude, we noticed this and that."*
This is what is fundamental. I shelter my responsibility. What distinguishes the signifier is here. I make a note of the sign as such. It's the acknowledgement of a receipt that is essential to communication insofar as it is not significant, but signifying. If you don't articulate this distinction clearly, you will keep falling back upon meaning that can only mask from you the original mainspring of the signifier insofar as it carries out its true function. (1993, 188)

For Lacan, the "subject's relation to his representation" is of fundamental importance (Leikert 2017, 660): how he locates himself within a network of enigmatic but potentially meaningful relations. The sea captain, in this extended metaphor, is more curious than he is anxious in the face of things "moving about in the night." And we notice his effort at location; he makes notes and indications, elements that constitute a system of mediation—in this case, a logbook—that allows the captain a degree of independence from the strange and enigmatic markings in the night sky.[13] Through the shaping of this event into a signifying system, the captain "shelters his responsibility" from the immediacy of impulsive reaction.[14] He has developed a way of representing himself and his place, a way of making himself, in other words, into an emerging human subject in relation to his perplexing surround. Lacan evokes something akin to Bion's emphasis on the subject's capacity to "alphabetize" or "think" about emotional experience, rather than be caught up (as certain higher primates, including humans, can be) in "all sorts of [automatic] displays."

The "original mainspring of the signifier" is a phrase to be taken (as is true with many of Lacan's locutions) literally. When he says "mainspring" he means to indicate a root element that has potential energy; it is something

---

[13] Again, one can see that Laplanche's (1999) influential concept about the "enigmatic signifiers from the other" is an extension of Lacan's basic insight.
[14] The classic Freudian example of mediation through signifiers is the "fort!–da!" story that is told in *Beyond the Pleasure Principle* (1920). I am grateful to Owen Hewitson for his help in parsing this passage from Lacan (personal communication).

central and potentially impactful. It is coiled and turns and releases like a spring. Consider Freud's "Dream of the Botanical Monograph" as an especially rich example of how a few key words, when "released," touch on the most intimate aspects of Freud's concerns at that moment: his history with cocaine and the death of a colleague, his writing the *Dream Book*, his sexual interest in a friend's wife, and the like (Freud 1900, 169–82). The signifier's potential energy rests in its inherently unanchored status, which allows free association to be relatively free, metaphor to be metaphoric, and the subject, as Ruti (2012) says, "to devise personally resonant forms of meaning" (52). These meanings resonate precisely because they are not fixed but are, instead, alive and open to further elaboration, as with our sea captain and his markings in the logbook.

In contrast to the logbook (or, more generally, any system of mediation) in which there are possible significations indicated by the markings that make it up, definitive facts can be facts only by way of brute experience, such as the ship running aground on rocks in shallow water. For the psychoanalyst, the "rocks" are "understanding" and "meaning," lures to be clearly illuminated so they can be more easily avoided. Definitive understanding, definitive meaning—these are fixed experiences and closed entities (what Lacan calls "significant" in the above quotation). They cease to be interpretable in the psychoanalytic sense; they just are.

It is important to reiterate, as with Bion, that we are talking about an ideal analytic position, a zero-point. From the perspective of this zero-point, the analyst's desire to understand and find meaning so as to tell the patient something about himself is, for Lacan, precisely the wrong kind of analytic desire. In such cases desire tips toward wish, signifier congeals into a signified. While the psychoanalyst may, even relatively routinely, offer "understanding and insight," from this ideal position of analytic desire such offerings are always inherently partial, lacking, and open to further elaboration, including the patient's utter disregard of what has just been offered. One can hear resonances in Lacan's warning about "understanding the patient" with Bion's concept of –K, the putting to use of knowledge in order not-to-know, in order to foreclose new experience, or in order not-to-experience something more enlivening, or unsettling, confusing, or painful.

In addition to having a sophisticated theory of the signifier-as-open-potential, Lacan had a clear statement that psychoanalysis is fundamentally a speech-relation. The signifier is the very grounding for the development of the unconscious as well as for the psychoanalytic method, a method that cures through speech. Crucially, speech is the articulation of desire; the signifier, especially within the context of the transference, is the carrier of human desire.[15] While Bion hoped somehow to move the analyst beyond language and used terms such as *reverie*, *intuition*, and *mystic* in an attempt to capture this particular position of analytic desire, Lacan sent the analyst on a journey *into* language, into not only its structuring conditions for the human subject but also all its rough edges, its echoes, its quietude, its senselessness and materiality.

## Objects of Analytic Desire

I have been arguing—Bion's famous admonition about desire notwithstanding—that he and Lacan share a similar perspective on the ideal position of the analyst within the clinical encounter. What is confusing, perhaps, in making this comparison is that for Lacan the immediate object of the analyst's desire is clearly different from Bion's. As I have described in the previous sections, Bion tended to bracket language so something unconscious might emerge, usually registered first in the analyst (the result, from a Bionian point of view, of projective identification). Lacan dove right into language for the same exact reason: that something unconscious, something unrealized, might be realized within the clinical moment.

"Intuiting emotional experience," for Bion, is central to the analyst's position and task. This is the proper object of analytic desire. Bion wished to minimize the analyst's reliance on conscious awareness ("sense impressions"), as well as on specific wishes (e.g., the end of the session, therapeutic gain) in order for an unconscious communicative experience of the emotional reality of the session to emerge. The "at-one-ment" that Bion speaks of is, as Ogden (2015) describes it, analogous to waking dreaming:

> When we dream—both when we are asleep and when we are awake—we have the experience of sensing (intuiting) the reality of an aspect of our unconscious life, and are at one with it. Dreaming ... is a transitive verb. In dreaming, we are not dreaming about something, we are dreaming something, dreaming up an aspect of ourselves. ... While dreaming, we are intuiting (dreaming up) an element of our unconscious emotional lives, and are at one with it in a way that differs from any other experience. (294)

---

[15] This is why, in part, Lacan repeatedly stressed that the analytic surface is not superficial; the wavelike movement of the patient's speech, animated by the transference, is desire.

Ogden is pointing us toward the immediacy of the reality of the unconscious that shows itself in dreaming (or in the analytic session), if the analyst has a freely mobile imagination at her disposal. Like the sea captain's, the analyst's capacity to imagine is a direct consequence of giving herself over to a process that is larger than she alone. If the analyst is overly anxious, concerned with surviving and maintaining a certain position, then the reality of something new showing itself will be foreclosed. "The analyst must engage in an act of self-renunciation," Ogden advises, so as to be in a position to be open to this kind of analytic experience (2015, 294).

Ogden gives clinical examples in which the analyst freely associates to what can only be called "sense impressions."[16] Here are two: "I sensed, when I met Ms. C in the waiting room, that she wanted to tell me that she genuinely loved her child" (298), and "When I opened the door to the waiting room, it seemed more starkly furnished than I'd remembered it" (302). With these impressions in tow, Ogden waits, listens, and sees what "comes up" in his experience ("dreaming the session") as he listens to his patient. Ogden's clinical illustrations, given to us in a paper about Bion, involve a sense of traversal, a moving through or over difficult and opaque territory until a clearing is in view. Eventually, something emotionally intense is clarified and shared between him and his patient. I take Ogden's description of his work to be useful information about the nature of Bion's "objects of analytic desire" (since Bion himself gives few detailed clinical examples to speak of).

For Lacan, intuition is too faulty a compass for the analyst to depend on. In fact, Lacan was deeply skeptical of intuition as a reliable analytic tool because of how easily the analyst can mistake her felt experience for the patient's.[17] While Lacan would entirely agree with the "self-renunciation" advocated by Ogden, for Lacan intuition is much too "self" and not enough "renunciation." Here is Lacan from an early paper, "The Function and Field of Speech and Language in Psychoanalysis" (1953), in which he bemoans the trend in psychoanalysis away from the structuring conditions of the Symbolic and the speech relation and toward the vagaries of experience, feeling, and emotional contact:

> Now all speech calls for a response ... there is no speech without a response, even if speech meets only with silence, provided it has

---

[16] In other words, Bion's attempt to move the analyst's capacities for attention beyond the senses is, practically speaking, impossible. Again, we are dealing with the aspirational and the asymptotic.

[17] I discussed this issue in detail in Chapter 3 in relation to the Imaginary register and the narcissistic basis of ego functioning.

an auditor. This is the heart of its function in analysis. But if the psychoanalyst is not aware that this is how speech functions, he will experience its call all the more strongly; and if emptiness is the first thing to make itself heard in analysis, he will feel it in himself and he will seek a reality beyond speech to fill the emptiness. This leads the analyst to analyze the subject's behavior in order to find in it what the subject is not saying.[18] (2002, 206)

And:

Nothing could be more misleading for the analyst than to seek to guide himself by some supposed "contact" he experiences with the subject's reality. This vacuous buzzword of intuitionist and even phenomenological psychology has become extended in contemporary usage in a way that is thoroughly symptomatic of the ever-scarcer effects of speech in the present context of psychoanalytic practice. (210)

Here we see an essential way in which Lacan differs from Bion. Both are keenly interested in what is emerging now in the session. But for Lacan the now-moment is always within the speech relation in which the movements of the signifier are animated by desire. Thus, the object of the analyst's desire is the *signifier-moment*—an opening, a half-saying, a turn, an inflection, in the patient's (or analyst's) discourse within this dialogic relation. These moments are intimately related to how the analysand is putting his or her world together. Already in 1953, Lacan critiques, more rightly than wrongly in my view, a gathering movement within psychoanalytic practice toward an emphasis on phenomenological experience and emotional "contact" at the expense of the speech-relation and the subject's relationship to his or her ways of self-representation.[19]

---

[18] Notice that Lacan offers a theory of countertransference as caused by an anxious identification on the part of the analyst, in this case an identification with an "emptiness"—enigma, strangerness—that is constitutive of the dialogic encounter that is psychoanalysis. The analyst's mirroring here is a telling consequence of the ways in which the analyst sees herself as a full presence (needing to be "in contact"), which limits her capacity to inhabit a position of lack and desire—a point discussed in Chapter 7.

[19] This critique is, as many readers know, more extensive than I have described here. Lacan is also criticizing the tendency of some analysts to reduce an analytic situation that is structured on the speech/dialogical relation to a simple re-creation of the mother–infant dyad, and which turns the analyst into a stand-in for the mother.

## The Analyst as Listening-Accompanist

If there is something both compelling and vague, on the one hand, about Bion's picture of psychoanalytic engagement, there is, on the other hand, something overly rigid and constraining in Lacan's bracketing of the phenomenological/experiential aspects of the analytic encounter.[20] After all—and this is a crucial point—*anything* that reaches the analyst's awareness while engaging with a patient in psychoanalysis can, in principle, take on the status of a signifier. A vague sense of unpleasure, a phrase or image that suddenly pops to mind, a feeling of despair or sadness, a ray of sunshine through the consulting room window—any of these (and countless other) moments of experience can, if registered as *potentially significant*, pose the same kinds of questions as those raised by a patient's dream or parapraxis or long silence.

With this broader conception of the signifier firmly in view, here is one way to fashion a picture of the analyst's desire in light of the ideas of Bion and Lacan I have been discussing here: fundamentally, the psychoanalytic session is structured on the speech-relation; the patient speaks and the analyst listens. This relation is both mutual and asymmetric, because the analyst is in a position of caretaking in relation to the patient. Within this basic dialogical structure, the analyst desires to isolate in the here and now registered (i.e., felt, heard, seen) signifiers (i.e., words and other sounds, facial indications, bodily movements, eye glances, images, feelings, silences, and the like) that point to *something more and potentially important that might be said*. These are indications and signals from the patient (and sometimes the analyst) that may require a comment, an accent or reinflection, forms of emphasis and punctuation from the analyst. An analyst can feel the mutuality of experience, the in-mixing of subjectivities and the sharing of space, and a kind of rhythmic call-and-response. Something is being created, rather than discovered, in this live, moving, diachronic engagement. But the asymmetry of the relationship is never elided. And if "meaning" and "understanding" are lures to be avoided, lest the dialogue shut down and emotional experience stagnate, this in no way means the patient's (or analyst's) speech is not an intimate part of this embodied dialogical dance. On the contrary, it is the analyst's responsibility to engage with the patient's speech-in-time, as it comes ready-to-hand, present, palpably aural and physically impactful. Bion's "undifferentiated zone" beyond the caesura of language must, in the end, find representation, whether through "direct discourse" or alive metaphor (Markman 2015). Intuitive moments, then, become signifying moments, as

---

[20] In the terms I used in Chapter 2, Lacan wishes to bracket key features of matricial space.

the analyst answers movement with movement, gesture with gesture, within a common rhythm (Muller 2016).

This analytic way is a kind of *listening-accompaniment*: at choice points the analyst intervenes within the rhythm of a series of nows, within the diachronic unfolding of the patient's speaking and experiencing ... *here* ... and ... ... *here* ... And ... ... ... (here). How the analyst knows that a point is "choice" is complex, but the point in question is one that *allows a question*, or calls for a response in the hope of furthering the opening of something potentially emotionally important or disturbing or enigmatic to the patient and often to the analytic couple. While rhythm and pace are key, so are the silences that form the "dark energy" surrounding the various soundings the patient makes (words, sighs, grunts, cries, giggles, and the like).[21] "The unconscious is what closes up again as soon as it has opened, in accordance with a *temporal pulsation*," Lacan stressed repeatedly in Seminar XI ([1964] 1981, 125, emphasis added). It is a question, then, of the analyst not missing a beat, or rather not missing the opening, the gap in the fabric of the dialogue when such an opportunity is there for the taking. Such an opportunity may offer itself once an hour or once an analysis (hopefully not that infrequently!). There are no rules. Whether now or later, this opening, this gap, is the moment of the emergence of the potentially significant, which, let's be clear, may be painful, disturbing, even upending.

Whitney Balliett, jazz critic for the *New Yorker* magazine for many years, wrote a memorable essay on "Big" Sid Catlett, a drummer who played in the 1940s with Louis Armstrong and later with Dizzy Gillespie. Balliett's description of Catlett's playing captures its real-time flow, his way of engaging rhythm, timing, and accent that seems to me directly analogous to the position of the analyst as listening-accompanist. Here is Balliett:

> Catlett's accompanying had an unfailing freshness and authority. He made everything that went on in front of him sound new. "Wow, man, I never heard you play that before," he seemed to say to each instrumentalist. His wire brushes achieved a singular, graceful, padding effect at slower tempos and a precise, hurrying, relentlessly pushing effect at faster tempos. When he switched to drumsticks in mid-performance,

---

[21] Although Lacan would quickly jettison the term intersubjective that he sometimes used in the 1950s to describe his perspective, it is not without irony that his emphasis on the rhythm of the spoken word and the analyst's listening-accompanying position has been elaborated empirically by intersubjective/relational psychoanalysts such as Beatrice Beebe. Her careful work (2014) on gestural turn-taking (through both verbal exchanges and bodily movements) between mother and young infant is, in my view, directly relevant to this discussion. See also Jaffe and Feldstein's *Rhythms of Dialogue* (1970).

as he often did, it was dramatic and lifting. His library of accompanying techniques was endless. He used different cymbals behind different instruments—a heavy ride cymbal behind a trumpet; the high hat, its cymbals half-closed, behind a trombone; a Chinese cymbal, with its sizzling sound, behind a clarinetist. All the while, his left hand worked out an astonishing series of accents on the snare drum. (1976, 108)

"Wow, man. I've never heard you play that before" is American vernacular that feels, admittedly, foreign to both Bion and Lacan. Yet it captures best how I understand their basic effort: the analyst's desire is a desire for the new within the psychoanalytic session, vivified by the transferential field—for an ideal, vanishing point, for what has yet to exist, which does not at all mean a desire for anything illusory.

This analytic desire instantiates, through its practice, through its doing, a particular faith in the patient and in the psychoanalytic process. This faith is, perhaps, hard to specify, but it is about the kind of support that the "wow, man" comment demonstrates: an implicit "this is possible, you can do this." If there is friction and strife between analyst and patient, as there sometimes is, an implicit, or sometimes an explicit, "it's okay, we can do it. We can get through this" is in order and is a further expression of the analyst's desire in support of the analysis.

## The Ethical Unconscious

I have used the word *futural* to indicate the realm of analytic desire that is most felicitous to the process and is a kind of leaning forward, on the part of the listening-accompanist, into whatever happens next. This emergent, this next, *comes from nothing*, literally. It is the yet-to-be-experienced. This is why both Lacan and the later Bion desired to go beyond the "ontic," beyond the physically extant, into the realm of the yet-to-be-realized. From this point of view, the unconscious is nonsubstantive—it is decidedly not buried, repressed stuff that exists in a warded-off place. Nor is it an "unrepresented mental state."[22] It is, instead, "pre-ontological" and ethical. Lacan, again from Seminar XI, said: "The status of the unconscious, which ... is so fragile on the ontic plane, is ethical. In his thirst for truth, Freud says, *Whatever it is, I must go there*, because somewhere, this unconscious reveals itself" ([1964] 1981,

---

[22] This is a common phrase that one meets with in the contemporary literature, and space constraints prevent me from discussing the concept at any length. But on its face it is an oxymoron.

33). Here is Grotstein (1997) describing Bion's "Transformations in 'O'" in similar terms:

> Bion replaced Freud's concepts of the id, the unconscious, and the "seething cauldron" with an epistemic function that harkens back to the creative role of the unconscious in the construction of dreams and jokes. ... Bion revealed the ineffable matrix, the container beyond the container of our existence, the eternally unsaturated Void, one that undermines every deterministic certainty with a mocking transcending doubt.[23]

And elsewhere in the same paper Grotstein writes that Bion's picture of the unconscious as "creative" and "eternally unsaturated" is an effort to "transcend the positivistic certainty of psychoanalytic ontic determinism." The "epistemic function" that Grotstein describes involves the immediacy of the unconscious revealing itself (as in Ogden's account of "waking dreaming").

If an ethics essentially consists in judgments of our actions, both of their intention and their outcome, their result, then the epistemic function of which Grotstein speaks, leads directly to an ethical one: the analyst's engagement with what "can be known" involves the analyst in a desire to "be there," to be (at one) with this "unconscious revealing," to hear it, to receive it, and to further its becoming.[24] I believe that from the point of view I have been articulating in this chapter, both Bion and Lacan situate the analyst in this place of emergence: Lacan called it lack or the Real,[25] and Bion called it O. Again, this emergence of the next is an ideal point, partly because the emergent present is never entirely free from the past, and synchronic moments ("points") are always part of formal diachronic movement (think, again, of the jazz drummer accenting a given *something* as the music pushes ahead).

Something is made in psychoanalysis, but it is not substantial; it does not have mass, nor is it material. The analyst's desire is to occupy a place that is without substance—eternally unsaturated, void—and to act in that

---

[23] J. Aguayo, the noted scholar of Bion's and Grotstein's work, dates this text, which carries a 1997 copyright, to a presentation Grotstein gave in 2006. It was never formally published (personal communication).

[24] For more detailed discussions of questions regarding psychoanalytic ethics, action, and desire, see Lacan ([1959–60] 1992), Kirshner (2012), Lear (2012), Friedman (2012), and Wilson (2012). Regarding ethics, character, and the analyst's offer of analysis, see Kite (2016), Kattlove (2016), Morris (2016), and Chapter 8 here.

[25] There is much more to say about this point. Lacan specifically designated the analyst's lacking position as the place of the *objet a*. See Kirshner (2005) and Chapter 5 here for a discussion of the role of lack in the analytic process.

place as may be necessary. A wish, in the Freudian sense, has a direct object and so is structured around satisfaction. The analyst's desire is without an object in its positivity. When desire becomes fixed in the wish for a specific object relation or experience, it ceases to be desire as such. As I describe elsewhere in this book, especially in the next chapter, countertransference is based on unrecognized desire, and clinical impasses begin when the analyst's desire gets reified into specific wishes. Impasses yield when what had been hitherto out of awareness and, instead, enacted-in-action becomes an object of reflection, of engagement, as the analyst's desire gets "reengaged" (see also Racker 1957). Bion's admonition regarding desire and memory is actually about wishes that get in the way of the analyst's capacity to sense something new and emotionally meaningful in the moment. For Lacan, in the end, desire's object is desire itself, to be open to the "further open." This is the true place of the analyst's desire—a place of potentially transformative emergence. The analyst's desire is to mark this movement, this emergence.

It is important to reflect, if briefly, on ways in which both Bion's and Lacan's objects of analytic desire can become hardened into wishes, and at times into subtle and not-so-subtle demands on the patient, and so clog up the analytic process. *Intuition, reverie,* and the like can too easily lead the analyst to overvalue her own ideas and feelings and mistake them for the patient's experience. This risk is substantial and involves a conceptual confusion about the Imaginary register, and the narcissistic nature of the functioning of the ego (as I explained in detail in Chapter 3). In this case, desire solidifies too easily into wish, as the analyst may become fixed on the putative validity of an idea or the importance of maintaining a position. These moments amount to the analyst indulging in an extreme form of self-reliance—as happens when the analyst has lost a feel for her lacking position, temporarily suspending participation in the dialogical relation, including the asymmetrical conditions established by transference. The analyst, in this case, ceases to "shelter her responsibility" within a flexible yet structured analytic frame. The well-known Bionian question is a good one: when is a "selected fact" merely an "over-valued idea" (Britton and Steiner 1994). In my estimation, often it is very hard to tell. The analyst's openness to her own necessary limitations (i.e., her own lack) is the way forward to an engagement with something new, perhaps previously unimagined and unformulated.

Lacan's focus on the speech relation, I believe, at least has the advantage of epistemological immediacy: the words have been spoken and heard, the pace experienced, the gaps, hesitations, tone, and prosody felt. And yet Lacanian objects of desire are at no less risk of reification. Here I have in mind the fetishizing of the signifier narrowly defined as the sound of the word, as if a unilateral focus on the materiality of the patient's speech (puns and the like) is enough to make a difference for a given patient. It is often not nearly enough, and is at times (as I discussed in Chapter 2) an unfortunate distraction, or worse, an occasion for alienation, even trauma. In this quite limited psychoanalytic horizon in which the broader experiential surround is bracketed, the Symbolic becomes the last lure of the Imaginary, as the analysis risks turning into an exercise of further alienation without therapeutic impact.[26]

As I emphasized in Chapter 3, all analysts, as Laplanche has said, work "under the constant threat of narcissistic closure" (1999, 81), in which desire becomes reduced to wish and is overly invested by the analyst with narcissistic value. Bion and Lacan point us away from narcissistic closure, away from anxious "displays" of wish and action in the face of the enigmatic, and toward the shelter of newly emergent representations, new articulations, and new experiences.

---

[26] In Chapter 7 I describe in more detail some of the problematic rigidities of the Lacanian approach.

# 7

# Desire and Responsibility: The Ethics of Countertransference Experience

*This chapter is a further extension of the ideas I introduced and explored in Chapters 3, 4, and 5. There I discussed the role of narcissism and the ego (Chapter 3), desire and resistance (Chapter 4), and lack and the analyst's attitude (Chapter 5). Here I engage the question of desire and countertransference and situate this discussion within the context of the ethics of psychoanalytic practice.*

*The deep dissatisfaction we find in every psychology—including the one we have founded thanks to psychoanalysis—derives from the fact that it is nothing more than a mask, and sometimes even an alibi, of the effort to focus on the problem of our own action—something that is the essence and very foundation of all ethical reflection.*
—Jacques Lacan, The Ethics of Psychoanalysis

As a profession we have become wary of overly satisfied descriptions of patients' dynamics and structures of psychopathology. This wariness has been painfully earned, as too often and too easily psychoanalytic theory has, wittingly or not, been used as a vehicle (and in some hands a weapon) to marginalize or even demonize identifiable groups of people, most notably gay men and women, and also women more generally. Obviously, psychoanalytic thought and practice cannot help but be influenced by and suffused with the key tropes and memes at play in the cultural surround, though its professional ethos—the face it thinks it shows to the world—aspires to something more universal, like the search for the unvarnished truth about the human mind and human being untainted by the myriad contingencies and accidents of local life.

Regarding the specifics of clinical practice, our reluctance to opine about psychopathology is due to multiple factors, some of which include the lack of predictive value of such descriptions, their uncertain genesis in relation to putative developmental factors, and their post-hoc explanatory status. As I have already suggested, this reluctance is the effect of the legacy of what might feel to some to be an unearned authority, the authority to pronounce the nature of the pathology said to reside *in* the patient while sparing the analyst a similarly authoritative pronouncement.

Racker (1957) may have been the first prominent analyst to note this weighty irony:

> The first distortion of truth in "the myth of the analytic situation" is that analysis is an interaction between a sick person and a healthy one. The truth is that it is an interaction between two personalities, in both of which the ego is under pressure from the id, the superego, and the external world. (307)

Since Racker's time, an intersubjectivist-inflected, two-person psychology has replaced a predominantly objectivist, one-person psychology in most analysts' conceptualizations of the psychoanalytic process.

Even if a two-person psychology is an accurate umbrella term to convey the basic orientation of most psychoanalysts today, in the literature we have felt on safer ground, I think, by turning out gaze inward on the analyst's experience. The analyst's activity—what she says, how she thinks, how she acts and enacts—has become the central psychoanalytic preoccupation. The gulf between self and other, analyst and patient, seems more difficult to bridge than the gap between the analyst's own conscious self-assessments and whatever unconscious stirrings are active underneath. Consequently, we have witnessed an ever-growing and voluminous literature on the countertransference, enactment, and self-disclosure. It might appear that analysts have become quite one-person in their orientation to the analyst's internal world.[1]

Yet psychoanalytic writers have not abandoned the task of understanding the dynamics and struggles of analysands. Analysts remain as dedicated to the psychoanalytic understanding of their patients as ever. It seems uncontroversial to say that the analyst's desire to understand remains central to her reasons for action in analysis. But this project of understanding has been

---

[1] Certainly, the now substantial literature on the analytic field attempts to ameliorate any unfortunate weighting in one direction (the patient) or the other (the analyst). But the concept of the field is, in my estimation, of limited clinical value if the ultimate goal of analysis is the patient's emergence as a subject in his, her, or their own right. To argue this point responsibly would take many more pages than I have at my disposal in the present work.

smuggled in underneath the cover of analytic self-scrutiny. That is, through examination of her countertransference experience, broadly construed, the analyst comes to understand and know the analysand psychoanalytically.

In the end, analysts are no less interested in describing patients' struggles in psychopathological language (splitting, projection, omnipotence, and the like). It is just that we tend to further these interests by examining our own internal states—what it feels like to be with a given patient at a given moment in time—as a, perhaps the, central way forward in this project of understanding.

The analyst's desire to understand (as well as other psychoanalytic desires that motivate her responses and actions) rests uneasily within the larger context in which the question of the analyst's actions is embedded, because action necessarily involves the analyst in an ethical situation. In his seminar on ethics, Lacan defines the term thusly: "An ethics essentially consists in a judgment of our action" (1992, 311). In this statement, Lacan is following Aristotle in the *Nicomachean Ethics* (2004), with "judgment" meaning the practical reasoning (*phronesis*) that inheres in any human action taken in relation to a goal or aim. As I discussed most especially in Chapter 3, the analyst's quest for understanding—"connecting the dots"—runs certain risks, including serving the analyst's aims at the expense of the patient's subjective emergence.

Importantly, one cannot take one's action as an object of serious inquiry without already believing one is responsible as an agent for the action. In other words, an ethics of analytic practice confronts the analyst with deeply personal questions regarding responsibility and judgment in a desire to delimit the truth—to figure out, as we tend to say colloquially, "what is going on" with ourselves and with our patients. As is implied by the epigraph at the beginning of this chapter, there are important senses in which analytic theory, especially perspectives that emphasize the analyst's looking inward to understand the other, can mask our effort to focus on the problem of our own action.

The word countertransference suggests directly that the analyst is responding to an outside stimulus—she is countering the patient's transference communication. The implication is that the analyst's action is a re-action, an action "again," following the action of the patient. Already one can sense the shrouding of the issue of the analyst's agency—and the desire that animates this agency—in the root elements of the word countertransference itself. The psychoanalytic origins of the term are well-known and reinforce this point: Freud coined the term in a letter to Jung (June 7, 1909) regarding the possibly erotic nature of Jung's relationship with Sabina Spielrein (McGuire 1974). Freud advised Jung "to dominate" his countertransference. The source of Jung's problem came from Miss Spielrein.

No doubt psychoanalysis has come a far distance since 1909. Consistent with the writings of Ogden (1994), Ferro (2002), Baranger, Baranger, and Mom (1983), and many others, analysts today tend to emphasize that the countertransference is an inextricable element in an interactional field constituted by transference and countertransference. For some analysts, any feeling or fantasy about a patient—any reaction of any kind—tends to be called "countertransference." Such a broadly construed notion of countertransference struggles to have even a modicum of standing within psychoanalytic clinical theory. If "everything" the analyst thinks and feels is countertransference, then nothing is.

Others, such as Renik (1993a), assert that the term countertransference should be retired as misleading, because all the analyst's reactions emerge from an irreducibly personal and subjective position. This view is akin to that expressed in the enactment literature regarding the inevitability of the analyst's expression through action of wishes and conflicts about which she has been unaware. In light of such an accepting and capacious view of countertransference within the even broader umbrella of a two-person psychology, it may appear that the questions the countertransference poses have been put to rest.

I believe this is a misguided view. In this chapter, I define countertransference in relation to the analyst's experience of pleasure and unpleasure (Faimberg 1992)—moments in which the analyst experiences a rise in tension, a feeling that something is "wrong" or "off." I want to limit the scope of countertransference to the analyst's experience of pleasure and unpleasure because it is through the analyst's experience of these feeling states that we can begin to clarify the ways in which the analyst's desiring position underwrites these states. In the literature on countertransference, the analyst's position as a desiring subject who wants specific experiences moment-to-moment in the work tends to be undertheorized, if not ignored altogether. Instead, we read about the varieties of the analyst's participation, influenced and constrained by his anxieties, history, internal object relations, and theory (Purcell 2004). Yet I think that most of these factors, however important they may be in influencing how we listen and what we do as analysts, are not, upon reflection, particularly specific in penetrating the nature of countertransference experience and clarifying our activity in the moment-to-moment process of clinical work.

"Irreducible subjectivity" is a general notion, as is "internal object relations." And "unconscious conflicts" born of the analyst's history tend to live at a considerable distance from the analyst's activity at any given moment. Further, soliciting the past to explain the present can have the feel of speculation, however earnest and honest such speculation may be. Such speculation, in fact, can obscure more relevant and impactful desires that motivate the analyst's activity in the trenches of a clinical hour. The analyst's theory, on the other hand, often has more direct impact on the analyst's state of mind and the conditions she imposes on the patient that can lead to an experience of unpleasure.

As a core, irreducible unit of measure, the analyst's desire—I have in mind her psychoanalytic desires—remains both insufficiently appreciated and insufficiently studied. This desire is often manifested in specific conscious or preconscious wishes that, when frustrated, become potentially accessible to the analyst. Schafer (2009) writes:

> The analytic literature amply explains the patient's role in becoming a frustrating object. Waiting to be sorted out are the needs of the analyst that are not being met; more exactly, these needs have been insufficiently analyzed in the context of the analyst's vulnerability to feeling frustrated. (75)

I contend that countertransference experience rests on the analyst's desire as it is engaged within the clinical encounter. The rest of this chapter amounts to an extended argument why this is so.

As the reader by now can appreciate, desire itself can be conceptualized in a number of ways, and in the pages of this book it has taken on somewhat different aspects. For the purposes of this chapter on countertransference let's posit the following: Unconscious desire arises from ontological conditions— the loss of our primary objects, the intercession of language, culture, and the law (i.e., the oedipal situation writ large) that create conditions in which we live as subjects. These conditions not only allow for but also require symbolic capacities (representation, memory, imagination, fantasy, and hope). This foundational desire is born of a fundamental lack.

While I will allude in this chapter to this fundamental and bedrock human desire born of lack, for the most part I am interested in desire's more experience-near derivatives. By this I mean the intentions, aims, and values that motivate our actions, especially our actions as analysts in the consulting room that have demonstrable impact on the analysand and the process. In general, the desires I am interested in are not deeply unconscious or shot through with the heavy residue of unresolved conflict.[2] Instead, I will focus

---

[2] Experience-near, preconscious desires may, of course, be fed by unconscious sources, but the connections between one and the other are often obscure and of variable relevance to the analyst's experiences of pleasure and unpleasure (i.e., countertransference). Certainly, analysts are often involved in longer-term, unconscious engagements that only become clearer over time, as I describe in the case of Byron later in this chapter.

on the more immediate desires that amount to the analyst's wanting specific experiences with a patient in the real-time work of analysis.

In this chapter, I wish to accomplish three things.

1. Theoretical: Establish that countertransference experience is dependent, necessarily, upon the particular desiring state of the analyst at that moment of experiencing and arises *logically prior* to other factors involving the patient.
2. Clinical: Describe the central importance of the analyst's taking her desire as a unit of measure and as the first order of business in unpacking her countertransference experience.
3. Ethical: Show how the analyst's desire and the countertransference experience that unfolds as a result of this desire are embedded in an ethical field in which responsibility, judgment, and truth are always in play, and the analyst and patient's sanity are at stake.

I orient myself to the question of the role of desire and countertransference via the "wider" countertransference perspective that is usually associated with the writings of contemporary Kleinians, such as Joseph, Feldman, and Spillius, among others. I enter into the conversation here because theirs is a strong and highly influential reading of the value of the analyst's countertransference experience. I take the phrase strong reading from the literary scholar Harold Bloom (1975): "A strong reading is one that itself produces other readings ... it must insist upon its own exclusiveness and completeness, and it must deny its partialness and its necessary falsification" (50).[3]

This strong, robust reading of the value of the analyst's countertransference allows me to then introduce a discussion of the analyst's desire. It was both Lacan ([1948] 2002; [1949] 2002), as early as 1936 with his original paper on the "Mirror Stage," and Racker (1957, 1968), in his remarkably prescient series of papers in the 1950s on countertransference, who discerned the fundamental role that the analyst's desires and wishes have in the clinical encounter. They both described in detail the hazard that unfolds if the analyst

---

[3] A further explication by Bloom (1975) is edifying: "We do not speak of poems as being more or less useful, or as being right or wrong. A poem is either weak and forgettable or else strong and so memorable. Strength here means the strength of imposition. A poet is strong because poets after him must work to evade him. A critic is strong if his readings similarly provoke other readings. What allies a strong poet and a strong critic is that there is a necessary element in their respective misreadings. But again I hear the question: 'Why do you insist upon a misreading?' My answer is that a reading, to be strong, must be a misreading, for no strong reading can fail to insist upon itself" (66). Obviously, I myself run the risk of misreading the wider countertransference view through my own "strong reading" of it.

does not take account of what she wants from the patient at any given moment. Racker's law of the talion and Lacan's dual relation describe a structure of dyadic relating that occurs when the analyst resists this accounting. In this resistant state the analytic gyroscope sits motionless, as the analyst's futural, anticipatory position is frozen in place.

I will describe the features of this structure of relating later in the chapter; for now, the reader should know that the talion law/dual relation involves a dyadic analytic field characterized by paranoia (often subtle), aggression/retaliation, and compliance/rebellion (as a third term is necessarily excluded). I consider the logic and importance of the theory of projective identification to the wider countertransference view, and that an appreciation of the talion law/dual relation renders problematic (to put it charitably) a wholesale acceptance of its logic and importance.

Finally, I move to the question of the ethics of countertransference experience. Taking my lead from Lacan's (1992) ethics of desire and Jessica Benjamin's (2004) concept of the moral third, I describe, via a clinical example, the ethical burdens that fall upon the analyst in light of her desiring position, and the serious consequences for the patient that depend on how the analyst handles these burdens.

Throughout this chapter, as is true of my overall effort in this book, I indulge the hope that it is possible to mix and compare theoretical models to felicitous and generative purposes, and to bring together seemingly disparate terms in an intellectually responsible way. Part of this responsibility is to represent faithfully, as best one can, a point of view with which one has disagreements. Further, comparative psychoanalytic scholarship must be willing, as I am here, to describe a landscape in which contrasts are as worthy to lay bare as are comparisons and similarities. In other words, *not all models are additive; some are incommensurable*. I intend to make these theoretical complexities clearer as the chapter unfolds.

## The "Wider" View of Countertransference and Projective Identification

Freud, as we know, viewed the countertransference as something the analyst should mitigate, if not altogether defeat. Klein, as I will describe later on, felt similarly. They share what has been called the "narrow" view of countertransference. They hold the minority perspective on the subject, as it is nearly settled doctrine in contemporary psychoanalysis that the countertransference is of crucial importance in the analyst's understanding of the patient's unconscious communications and conflicts. Heimann (1950), in her groundbreaking paper, stated the case with authority: "The analyst's countertransference is not only part and parcel of the analytic relationship, but it is the patient's *creation*, it is part of the patient's personality" (83, italics in original).

Several seminal analytic thinkers, such as Bion, Segal, and Joseph, have extended and deepened Heimann's basic idea. According to Spillius (Spillius and O'Shaughnessy 2012), "most British analysts have adopted the wider definition of countertransference advocated by Paula Heimann and others rather than the narrower definition of Freud and Klein" (53). The wider view in contemporary psychoanalysis is captured in canonical statements such as this one by Joseph (1985):

> Much of our understanding of the transference comes through our understanding of how our patients act on us to feel things for many varied reasons; how they draw us into their defensive systems; how they unconsciously act out with us in the transference, trying to get us to act out with them; how they convey aspects of their inner world built up from infancy … which we can often only capture through the feelings aroused in us, through our countertransference, used in the broadest sense of the word. (447)

In this wider view, the countertransference is the result of the patient's induced disturbance of the analyst's mind. Therefore, as Eagle (2010) writes, from this perspective, "the countertransference virtually always serves as a guide to knowledge about the patient's mental states" (220).

Projective identification as a psychoanalytic concept has its own complex history. For my purposes the term refers to the putative happening in which the patient "makes" or "pressures" the analyst to feel or do things that she experiences as alien and unwanted. The analyst's experience of unpleasure, in other words, is caused by the patient via this projective, identificatory, and unconscious process. The deep penetration of the theory of projective identification into the clinical thinking of a large and disparate group of analysts has given ballast to the wider view of countertransference. Over time, in fact, projective identification has itself taken on "wider" implications. With Bion's extension of the concept into the routine of mother–infant interactions, projective identification, rather than being seen as an unusual and pathological mechanism, is now regarded by many as an essential feature of mental functioning and as an important means of communicating emotional states. Projective identification has come to be viewed normatively, as a kind of "psychological breathing" (Wollheim 1993).

Here is the basic story of projective identification in the clinical setting from the wider countertransference perspective. If a patient wishes to be rid of "parts" (feelings, ideas, phantasies) of himself that are felt to be noxious or threatening, then one way to do so is to use the analyst as a place to put these parts. The analyst registers this impact by way of her subjective sense of dis-ease and unpleasure. For example, the patient unconsciously projects a fantasy of a sado-masochistic object relationship onto the analyst; consequently, the analyst feels pressured to act critically or submissively—that is, to conform with the felt pressure or to resist it. Even here things are not very clear: does the analyst simply feel "angry" at the patient (with accompanying conscious reveries of critical thoughts or images of harming the patient), or does the analyst feel "pressured" to be angry at the patient? The former is a direct, first-person experience, the latter is already an inference regarding the source and cause of this experience. In any case, if the analyst is feeling dis-ease, it may seem reasonable to assume that the patient has engendered this feeling in the analyst. Further (and this is crucial for our understanding of the power of the wider countertransference view), it is incumbent upon the analyst to investigate her countertransference because it is the most reliable and direct access the analyst has to the unconscious of the patient (the contours, that is, of the patient's internal object relations and transference).

Many (e.g., Feldman 1997; Steiner 2011) have written of the necessity of a fertile ground in the analyst in which the patient's projections can germinate; this is the way the countertransference can be felt by the analyst. Also, in working through the countertransference (Brenman-Pick 1985), the analyst gains experiential knowledge about the specific object relationship the patient has projected by containing and thinking about this experience (Bion 1970)—and, possibly, may be moved to interpret aspects of this experience to the patient in words that refer to the patient's expectations, wishes, and anxieties. Given many patients' struggles with meaningful change, for the analyst this is difficult, repetitive, and often painstaking work.

In the wider countertransference perspective, informed by the theory of projective identification, the analyst tends to work by way of analogy, as if to say: "If this dynamic is going on in me, it is likely going on in the patient, but it's too painful for the patient to know it. He needs me to know it so I can name it, describe it, for him."[4] This analogical way of working is important to recognize, and I will discuss it in more detail later in the chapter.

---

[4] There is an implicit ethical principle at play here: through the countertransference, the analyst makes "contact" with the most intimate aspects of the patient's psyche. If the analyst shies away from using countertransference in this fashion, she is avoiding the most difficult and fundamental conflicts with which the patient struggles.

## The Narrow View of Countertransference

Analysts know that the wider view of countertransference is not without risk. Why else would it be routinely accompanied by the recommendation, like a kindly and protective chaperone, that the analyst must, as Bion said, "differentiat[e] the patient's contribution from his own"? (Spillius 1988, 32). One finds this piece of seemingly reassuring advice repeated throughout the countertransference literature. Racker (1957), for example, specifies that, through an internal "division" (309), a form of self-analysis unfolds in which the analyst observes his experience, takes it as an object, and so gains distance from it. This allows the analyst to clarify relative contributions from himself and from the patient.

Money-Kyrle (1956) emphasizes similarly: when the analyst "feels burdened" by the patient, she must "become conscious of the phantasies within him, recognize their source, separate the patient's from his own, and so objectify him [the patient] again" (363). Spillius (1992) averred that analysts may easily confuse their own feelings with those of the patient, and that ongoing psychological work by the analyst is necessary to differentiate feelings that originate in the patient from those that originate in the analyst.

Feldman (1997) captures more of the bidirectional nature of projective mechanisms in the course of an enactment. He specifically describes a "pressure towards identity" that the patient and the analyst exert on each other, by attempting to bring into harmony the "pre-existing phantasies that partly reassure or gratify, and those with which [patient and analyst are] confronted in the analytical situation" (229). Here Feldman emphasizes the difficulty the analyst may encounter between a preferred view of the self and the role the analyst believes she is expected to play in a given clinical moment. The analyst, through a mixture of internal work and endurance, emerges on the other side in a somewhat recovered position as analyst, separated from the patient's "pressure." Feldman writes:

> The analyst's temporary and partial recovery of his capacity for reflective thought rather than action is crucial for the survival of his analytical role. The analyst may not only feel temporarily freed from the tyranny of repetitive enactments and modes of thought himself, but he may believe in the possibility of freeing his patient, in time. (1997, 239)[5]

---

[5] Feldman intuits the problem, but without the added help of a more robust theory of the ego, narcissism, and the hazards of bias and the dual relation, the analyst, as I go on to explain, remains in a clinically and ethically compromised position. This chapter is precisely about how the analyst "frees" herself from the dual-relation/talion law dynamic.

While the details of this internal work of differentiation and recovery are often described with great care, upon examination it remains hard to put embodied experience to nouns like internal division, phantasies, source, and capacity, along with the accompanying transitive verbs become, separate, recognize, and free. How does one go about the job of parsing relative contributions to one's countertransference? How do I differentiate the patient's feelings, attributions, and pressures from those that originate in me? When, in other words, is a "narrow" countertransference (the source of which is thought to be the analyst's unconscious desire and conflict) lurking in what seems to be a wider countertransference experience (the source of which is the patient, via projective identification)?

To sort this out is anything but a straightforward project. In reality, it is often difficult for the analyst, caught in a strong countertransference experience, to know where to start. At times, in fact—and as if in response to the true difficulty I am describing—caution regarding the analyst's contribution to the countertransference is given parenthetically, as if an obligatory mention is all that's needed, as if, that is, it nearly goes without saying. For example, Sodré, in a deep and comprehensive paper on projective identification, says between parentheses:

(I am of course taking it for granted that, as the analyst, one must always try to differentiate between what is being projected and the effect this has on oneself, which is due at least partly to one's own psychological make-up.) (Sodré quoted in Spillius and O'Shaughnessy 2012, 145)

The parsing of countertransference experience is arguably *impossible* if there is a significant gap in our theoretical understanding of its nature. And if the nature of countertransference experience is obscure, then our technical handling of it will be wobbly at best and will have significant clinical and ethical consequences. So I now turn to investigating the role of the analyst's desire in establishing necessary conditions for countertransference to emerge as such.

## The Analyst's Basic Desiring Position

It is obvious that analysts want things in and from their work, and want things from their patients. (Note, for example, in the foregoing quotation from Feldman, the author's desire to recover his position as a functioning analyst who can think and reflect.) This point may seem prosaic and anodyne. But in fact, like Poe's purloined letter, the analyst's desire as expressed in specific wishes, aims, and values is out in the open, right under our very noses, though often enough it remains bracketed by parentheses, unseen and unexamined. In descriptions of the psychological effort analysts are encouraged to make in grappling with their countertransference experiences, one cannot help but notice both an *overdescription* (consider the "many varied reasons" Joseph lists in the foregoing quotation), and at the same time a *lack of precision*, an indeterminacy at the heart of things. Maybe this vagueness is unavoidable. After all, our figurative language can only go so far in describing experience, especially experience that is said to be based on nonverbal communication and impact. Further, some might say that our experience of countertransference is the end result of compromises and necessarily serves multiple functions (Waelder 1936).

And yet this lack of precision suggests a wish not to look further. Or perhaps it suggests an effort to look everywhere (i.e., the patient's conflicts/fantasies/projections, and the analyst's conflicts/fantasies/projections) except at the irreducible element that underwrites the entirety of the analyst's activity. The analyst's desire gives foundational support to all that she does, including experiencing what we call countertransference. Analysts write about being made to feel pressured, frustrated, worried, or curiously oversatisfied or comfortable in a given clinical moment. Feeling these feelings and noticing them rest on the analyst's being in a state of desire.

The analyst's desire is always already at play, from the moment she opens the office, turns on the lights, and greets the first patient of the day. This desire puts the analyst, by definition, in a position of lack relative to the Other—not only the patient as "other," but also the Other as instantiated in the analyst's ideals and unconscious, as well as internal representations of her colleagues and the profession.

Racker (1957) wisely notes the position in which the analyst finds herself due to a desire that is perhaps *the* analytic desire, that is, the analyst's "wanting to cure":

> The analyst communicates certain associations of a personal nature even when he does not seem to do so. These communications might begin, one might say, with the plate on the front door that says Psychoanalyst or Doctor. What motive (in terms of the unconscious) would the analyst have for wanting to cure if it were not he that made the patient ill? In this way, the patient is already, simply by being a patient, the creditor, the accuser, the "superego" of the analyst; and the analyst is his debtor. (325)

Racker is one of the few analysts whose clinical thinking one cannot do without. Here his description may feel extreme, perhaps, but it is not. He captures an important aspect of the basic working conditions of the analyst—a tough spot for the analyst to be in, to be sure, given the stakes typically involved. In this description, Racker expresses some of the "impossibility" inherent in what we do. But my emphasis here is a little different: this is Racker's unflinching, face-to-face recognition and acceptance of the analyst's basic desiring position—a position that is inevitable, unavoidable, and at times deeply troublesome.

Racker, as I have said, tackles the question of the analyst's desire head-on. But as a collective, we have tended to turn away, or at least not to theorize fully our own purposive, intentional involvement in our clinical work. Our discomfort with our desiring position involves, I believe, the intimate connection between desire and narcissism. Desire, in other words, smacks too much of "self-interest." As Cooper (2010) writes: "We fear the analyst's narcissism or self-interest because it is a potential threat to the analytic situation. But, it is also essential to understanding the patient's and analyst's sometimes malignant efforts to pretend that it is not there" (173).

We know as psychoanalysts that, if something is unacknowledged, it is all the more powerful for being so. The analyst's desire, if never spoken about, alluded to, whether taken for granted or entirely repressed, can only agitate and perturb the analytic process of which it is a part.

The analyst's desiring position is also the first place we ought to look in unpacking our countertransference experience. That is, by focusing on the analyst's desire, we can become much more precise about the methodology of differentiation, how the analyst actually goes about the work of separating her self and her self-interests from those of the patient. In seriously taking account of what she wants in the moment with the analysand—usually in retrospect and sometimes with trepidation—the analyst goes about inhabiting the architecture, the logic, of the countertransference. The analyst does this through real time, active living in that structure.

## The Logic of Countertransference Experience

As a way of entering into the logic of countertransference, let's start with a consideration of Melanie Klein's perspective. Klein's name is often mistakenly attached to a robust view of the clinical utility of countertransference; in fact, however, she remarkably is cautious about its epistemic and clinical value. As mentioned, hers, along with Freud's, is a narrower view of the countertransference.

As quoted by Spillius (2007), Klein cautions younger analysts to examine themselves first, before attributing to the patient what the analyst is feeling for reasons that might have little to do with the patient. Spillius reports Klein's comments from notes she had taken in weekly meetings Klein had in the last years of her life with the leading lights of the next Kleinian generation: Segal, Joseph, Bion, Spillius, Feldman, among others. In this rather auspicious context (one of the great moments in the history of psychoanalysis!), Klein's statements about countertransference are surprisingly forceful: "I have never found that the countertransference has helped me to understand my patient better. If I may put it like this, I have found that it helped me to understand myself better" (78).

Klein continues:

> At the moment when one feels that anxiety is disturbing one, I think probably it is again a matter of experience, one would really on the spot come to the conclusion what went on in oneself. Therefore, I cannot really find a genuine account that countertransference, though unavoidable, is to be a guide towards understanding the patient, because *I cannot see the logic of that*; because it obviously has to do with the state of mind of the analyst, whether he is less or more liable to be put out, to be annoyed, to be disappointed, to get anxious, to dislike somebody strongly, or to like somebody strongly. I mean it has so much to do with the analyst that I really feel that my own experience—and that goes back a very long time—that I had felt that—is rather to find out within myself when I had made a mistake ... and then I really found it was a difficulty in myself. (Klein quoted in Spillius 2007, 78, emphasis added)

Klein explains what she means by "I cannot see the logic of that" by referring to the "obvious" relationship of the analyst's state of mind and its liabilities to her experience of countertransference. "State of mind" and "liable" take us a few steps in the right direction, but they are not particularly precise. What we are really talking about are intentional mental states, most notably, *states of desire*. In what follows, I will set out this "logic" and demonstrate the role of the analyst's desire as a necessary condition in countertransference experience.

Countertransference begins with a state of dis-ease in the analyst. I mean dis-ease in the broadest possible sense. It might involve worry, anxiety, panic, confusion, or, less intensely, a wondering about a pleased or satisfied response to the patient.[6] Faimberg's (1992) notion of the analyst's countertransference position, a comprehensive description of the analyst's overall functioning, places at its center the problem of the analyst's unpleasure. This unpleasure,

---

[6] In other words, as Feldman (1997, 2007) notes, the analyst can feel dis-ease about having felt ease or satisfaction.

this dis-ease, is the signal that tells us—or perhaps compels us—to take this dis-ease as an object of self-questioning, and to grapple as best we can with the ways in which we are implicated in the creation of this experience.

*What does it mean to be in a state of unpleasure or dis-ease? It means I have a desire that is unsatisfied.*

Let's examine the basic structure of an intentional state to clarify this crucial point. Searle (1983) writes:

> Every intentional state consists of an intentional content in a psychological mode. Where that content is a whole proposition and where there is a direction of fit, the intentional content determines the conditions of satisfaction. Conditions of satisfaction are those conditions which, as determined by the intentional content, must obtain if the state is to be satisfied. (12–13)

Desires, as Searle describes, "cannot be true or false, but can be complied with, fulfilled or carried out, and ... they have a 'world to mind' direction of fit" (8). A desire is fulfilled or not depending on what happens in the world relative to the desire regarding those happenings; hence the "world to mind" direction of fit.

If we take a typical analytic desire as an example of what Searle is describing, we get something like the following:[7]

1. Analyst's desire: that the patient attempts to say whatever comes to mind. This is the specific intentional content of the desire. Notice that the intentional content is a representation of its conditions of satisfaction.
2. Conditions of satisfaction of the desire: that the patient in fact says whatever comes to mind.
3. If the patient is saying whatever comes to mind, then the analyst is satisfied. If the patient is not saying whatever comes to mind, then the analyst is not satisfied. To use Faimberg's (1992) expression, the analyst is in a state of unpleasure.

There are aspects of this formulation of intentionality—and of desire, specifically—that may strike some readers as fundamentally irrelevant to psychoanalysis. First, this formulation appears to describe conscious mental

---

[7] Clearly, one can list a number of common analytic desires: to "contain," to understand, to interpret, to have the patient listen to the interpretation, to help/cure, to be without memory and desire. Each of these desires has its own conditions of satisfaction.

experience, and psychoanalysis is the investigation of the unconscious. Second, its linearity and unidimensionality ring false. After all, we know that the mind is in conflict, and that conscious mental experience is a compromise of different forces, even different desires, including unconscious desires.

These two objections, while superficially compelling perhaps, do not cast doubt on our description of the basic structure of unpleasure. As I'll describe in some detail in the case examples to follow, *the analyst is often unaware that she had and continues to have a desire prior to her being in a state of dissatisfaction.* The desire had been only descriptively unconscious—or, more usually, preconscious—and it is only through internal psychological effort (a key element in Faimberg's broader description of the analyst's countertransference position) that the analyst works backward—*from conscious unpleasure to (the emerging into consciousness of) an unsatisfied desire.*

It is readily observable that many of the analyst's operative, impactful desires are accessible to consciousness. The countertransference literature tends to describe exactly these kinds of mental states. That is, even though it is often asserted that the analyst's countertransference struggles are related to unconscious fantasy, in fact the desires that do the impactful work (for want of a better description) have, often enough, an uncertain relationship to unconscious fantasy.

## Racker's Seminal Contribution

What I am describing is entirely consistent with Racker's (1957, 1968) pathbreaking work on countertransference. Some aspects of Racker's ideas have found a lasting place in the literature and in the thinking of many analysts, independent of theoretical stripe. I have in mind, for example, the notions of concordant and complementary identifications. But other contributions of Racker's have tended to be deemphasized or lost. These ideas have to do with the analyst's desires and what Racker calls the law of the talion ("an eye for an eye, a tooth for a tooth"). As Racker shows repeatedly in his clinical examples, the analyst's desire, when frustrated yet unrecognized, leads, via the talion law, to a collapse of the analytic space. In this collapse, one finds a concrete world of mutual projection, self-other confusion, paranoia, hostility, and retaliation. The patient is put in a position of alienation in relation to the analyst's desire, which the patient either complies with (usually via identification) or rebels against. These are moments of trauma for the patient.

As one example among many, Racker (1957) describes the first session of an analysis "in which a woman patient talks about how hot it is and other matters which to the analyst (a woman candidate) seem insignificant" (332). Straightaway one can see that the analyst has imposed conditions of satisfaction onto the patient and has found the patient's productions wanting. The analyst is dissatisfied—that is, she is in a state of desire. Racker continues:

> She says to the patient that very likely the patient dares not talk about herself. Although the analysand was indeed talking about herself (even when she was saying how hot it was), the interpretation was, in essence, correct, for it was directed to the central conflict of the moment. But it was badly formulated, and this was so because of the countertransference situation. For the analyst's "you dare not" was a criticism, and it sprang from the analyst's feeling of being frustrated in a desire; this desire must have been that the patient overcome her resistance. (332)

Racker explains further on: "What has happened? The patient's mistrust clashes with the analyst's desire for the patient's confidence; therefore, the analyst does not analyze the situation" (333).

Finally, Racker offers the following, broader conclusion:

> What makes these happenings so important is the fact that the analysand's unconscious is fully aware of the analyst's unconscious desires. Therefore, the patient once again faces an object that wishes to force or lure the patient into rejecting his mistrust, and that unconsciously seeks to satisfy its own desires or allay its own anxieties, rather than to understand and satisfy the therapeutic needs of the patient. (334)

The reader can appreciate the power of Searle's (1983) analysis of the structure of a desire, as quoted earlier, in relation to the case Racker describes. The analyst "desires the patient's confidence" and wants the patient to be "open" in a particular way that she is not. The analyst is dissatisfied (the conditions of satisfaction are not met). It is hard to call "the analyst's desire for the patient's confidence" an unconscious fantasy (though it may be a derivative of a fantasy); this desire is accessible to consciousness and is the impactful desire in the moment.

And here is the psychoanalytic rub: the dissatisfied party wishes to retaliate, to even the playing field, to "right a wrong."[8] The analyst then pressures the patient to comply with her desire (a world-to-mind direction of fit). Most important, the patient knows what the analyst wants, at least

---

[8] Here we have an example of the Sartrean cycle of "bad faith" and *ressentiment* I mentioned in the Preface.

unconsciously and often preconsciously (Hoffman 1983). The analyst's and patient's desires, as Racker says, "clash." In case after case, Racker shows us how the analyst stumbles over her own unacknowledged desire, as if she had tripped over a split in the sidewalk. Racker is highlighting a crucial aspect of analytic functioning and of the countertransference that is routinely described in the analytic literature but variably examined, if examined at all.

The analytic literature, at least as far as clinical theory goes, is filled with the kinds of cases Racker describes. I want to mention four cases as familiar, perhaps classic examples. Leclaire (1998) reports an analyst's faint uneasiness at his patient's description of a fantasy of stealing a painting from an art gallery and an item from the analyst's waiting room. This uneasiness leads the analyst to rehearse in his mind basic theoretical constructs such as castration, and to address, by insinuation (because the analyst is caught up in an anxious/desiring state of mind), the rivalrous nature of the patient's aggressive fantasies. Renik (1993b) grows irritated when his patient complains about his (the patient's) suffering. The analyst responds in a critical fashion and only retrospectively realizes that he was engaged in a suffering contest with his patient. Ogden (1997) reports: "My muscles tensed and I experienced a faint sense of nausea as I heard the rapid footfalls of Ms. B. racing up the stairs leading to my office" (164); the patient lies down and complains that the couch is uncomfortable. The analyst then makes a retaliatory interpretation, of which, to himself, he takes note. Feldman (2007) feels pressured to "join the patient" (238) in the patient's excitement in telling his analyst a story. The analyst tells the patient that he, the analyst, is meant to join him in this excited way, and the patient feels criticized. Notably, Feldman does not report to us whether he registered his own dissatisfaction (i.e., "feeling pressured" and his desiring state) prior to his interpretation to the patient. I will look more closely at this case later in this chapter.

These examples are merely representative of case reports in the literature in which the analyst is in a state of desire relative to the patient. In each of these vignettes, things proceed with difficulty and (as is often the way with case vignettes) end up reasonably well. But the analyst's desire as a unit of measure, as the place to look first as the source of countertransference, tends to be deemphasized, or is not acknowledged at all—and so it remains unexamined and, therefore, undisturbed. The nature of the countertransference, in which every discomfort experienced by the analyst implies a prior unsatisfied desire, remains obscure.

When this is the situation, the talion law is usually in play. One might be tempted to say that when the talion law is prominent, the analyst is in a state of resistance relative to the patient's speech. This may be one outcome, to be sure. But the essential point is that the analyst is in a state of resistance relative to her own desiring state of mind. This resistance is the analyst's; the patient did not "cause" it. As I will describe later on, the ethical implications of this burden are substantial and important to consider for the analyst's genuine engagement in the work and for the survival of the analysis.

To come full circle, I think we can better appreciate Klein's assertion that the countertransference "obviously" depends on the analyst's state of mind, which we can now specify as a particular state of desire. This does not mean, as I will describe in more detail later, that the countertransference begins and ends with the analyst's desire; it means that it begins with it, that it is the first place the analyst ought to look for its bedrock source. In this sense, the analyst learns about her own desire in the countertransference. I believe this is why Klein says that in examining her countertransference, she learns about herself, not about her patient.

## The Law of the Talion and the Dual-Relation Resistance

When frustrated or anxious or perhaps notably satisfied in the clinical moment, the analyst typically does not ask himself: what is it I am wanting from this patient that I am not getting? If the analyst is caught in an experience of unpleasure and is not exploring this question right off the bat, further problems ensue. I would like to explore, through a closer look at Racker's and Lacan's ideas, what can unfold if the analyst's unpleasure is not appreciated as a marker of her desire, and instead is believed, via analogical thinking, to be a mere reflection of the patient's struggle.

Racker and Lacan came from different psychoanalytic traditions, and there are significant contrasts in their overall conceptions of psychoanalysis. For example, Racker had a profound appreciation for the theory of internal object relations; Lacan did not. But on the basics of ego functioning, narcissism, aggression, and rivalry, they share much in common, especially from a clinical point of view.

Racker's perspective on the role of the talion law in clinical work is similar to Lacan's concepts of the Imaginary register and the dual relation (which I discussed in detail in Chapters 3 and 4). The dual relation/talion law is important for analysts to understand, because without it, the analyst, caught in a position of unpleasure and dissatisfaction, can "drown" in the countertransference. If the analyst remains unaware of the desire she wishes were satisfied—unaware, that is, of the pressure she is putting on the patient in terms of conditions of satisfaction—then there is a clash of desires, and a paranoid, mirroring interaction ensues. As Racker describes, this often leads to "a kind of paranoid ping-pong" (1957, 318) between analyst and patient. This interaction is traumatizing for the patient and disturbing to the analyst.

The dual relation/talion law is not just a question of metaphors, like ping-pong or like a "seesaw" (Aron 2006, 351). Racker and Lacan are describing an *anatomy* of relating that is dual/duel in nature.[9] Racker emphasized punishment and retaliation: an eye for an eye, a tooth for a tooth. Lacan stressed the origins of the ego in a mirroring relation with the mother that creates in the infant a mixture of narcissistic jubilation, incipient agitation, and misrecognition. In the dual relation, each party tends to see herself in the other and to measure the other on the basis of her measure of herself. Each party sees herself as a full presence. Hence, denials of lack, loss, and difference are structural tendencies of ego functioning. I call this "normal narcissism" (Wilson 2010).

Racker's appeal to the biblical law of the talion gives further dimensionality and scope to the narcissistic basis of the ego I explored in Chapter 3. Here are the key features of the talion law/dual relation that one finds at work in psychoanalysis:

1. Bidirectional attributions. That is, what the analyst believes the patient is doing to the analyst, the analyst is also doing to the patient.
2. A paranoid analytic field.
3. Feelings/affects tend to be reciprocated. Racker, for example, notes that a positive transference will be met with a positive countertransference and a negative transference with a negative countertransference.
4. When in a state of desire in relation to the other person, there is a strong tendency to "battle it out"—to "clash," as Racker (1957, 333) says. Thus, a latent aggressiveness lurks within the dual relation in which a contest of wills is enjoined, as well as a wish to retaliate (Lacan [1948] 2002). Each party insists that the other recognize her desire.

Of special note is that because the relation is dual, there is an inherent confusion of self and other, and there is no third position as a way to adjudicate "truth." Instead, the exercise of power (often subtle and unspoken) takes over, with compliance/submission or rebellion/domination its hallmarks, as Jessica Benjamin describes in her 2004 paper, "Beyond Doer and Done-To." When

---

[9] The Barangers' concept of the bastion is a kindred notion to the dual relation/talion law and shares many features with the structure described here (Baranger, Baranger, and Mom 1983).

caught in the grips of a dual-relation resistance, the analyst is necessarily not taking ownership of her desiring position. Because the analyst is not acknowledging her desire to herself, any manner of interpretation regarding the patient's unacknowledged motivation or warded-off wish only solidifies the structure of the dual-relation resistance. This basic point I investigated at length in Chapter 4.

The language I am using here is strong and appropriate when discussing impasses in analysis; impasses undoubtedly involve the dynamics of the dual relation/talion law and often carry a weighed-down, burdened, or crisis atmosphere. But there are more usual interactions and exchanges between analyst and patient in which the dual relation/talion law hovers in the background, or conditions the analytic field in ways that are subtle but no less important for the analyst to grasp. In some respects, it is easier for the analyst to consider her desire when embroiled in a significant impasse. This may prove more elusive in the usual, day-to-day interactions in which the analyst may have difficulty owning a desiring position. Cooper (2010) writes:

> Instances of analysts externalizing levels of responsibility onto the patient are far more common than we realize ... I find that in these circumstances the analyst wants the patient to yield to the analyst's interpretations to provide affirmation of the analyst. (148)

## The Wider Countertransference View in Light of the Dual Relation/Talion Law

Analytic work that takes place under the aegis of the wider countertransference perspective is often quite complex. Racker (and Faimberg 1992, who followed in his footsteps) describes in detail the ways in which the contours of the analyst's countertransference highlight, but do not necessarily replicate, the details of the patient's transference. That is, the analyst may feel unpleasure for reasons that touch on her own desires and conflicts. Even so, this does not mean that the patient's transferential struggles are not similar to what the analyst registers and works through in her countertransference. Sometimes they are, and sometimes they aren't.

Further, the analyst's specific difficulty experienced in the clinical moment may be a clue to what the patient is contending with. This is what Racker points to in his concept of complementary identification: the analyst is identifying with an unwanted aspect of the patient's inner experience (i.e., a projected internal object) and so feels angry or protective or anxious, etc.

Or, the analyst feels that she is "expected" to react in a specific manner and finds herself "wanting" to act in this way.

Yet, as we have seen from examining the dual relation/talion law in detail, the analyst's expectations are always embedded within the patient's expectations as experienced by the analyst. As Racker strongly implies in his work, if the analyst can clarify her own desire that is admixed in the identification or the feeling of pressure, then she may be in a better position to describe to the patient an important aspect of the patient's struggle at that moment. But within the wider countertransference view, the desire of the analyst has an uncertain status. In my reading of the literature, I have yet to find a clear statement on the matter and am led to believe that the wider countertransference view, underwritten by the enthusiastic embrace of projective identification, does not have any place for the analyst's desire as a central aspect of the psychoanalytic process. If this is the case, then it would be difficult for the analyst to grasp the nature of her countertransference experience and to attempt to distinguish her own contribution from that of the patient.

As an instance of the complexity of the matter of the analyst's desire, the dual relation, and countertransference, let's look more closely at the case described by Feldman (2007) to which I previously alluded. It is true, of course, that I am using Feldman's case for purposes other than he intended; yet it seems to me crucial that our clinical literature serves more than a simple illustrative function. Ideally, it should be the locus of healthy and respectful debate. The clinical information Feldman provides is an especially suitable opportunity to read material that is informed by the wider countertransference view through the lens of the dual relation/talion law.

Let's recall that Feldman wishes to demonstrate the ways in which the patient projects an unconscious object relationship onto the analyst, pressuring the analyst to respond in a manner that reinforces the status quo ante. The patient, Mr. G, begins the first session after a summer holiday by expressing a worry about talking with the analyst, and saying that "he feared that what he brought up might not be serious enough, or that he would simply describe the events and experiences of the holiday in a way that would not prove useful" (2007, 788). Feldman continues: "He was very concerned about what kind of patient he was, and whether he could speak to me in a way I would be interested in, value, and find helpful" (788).

Analysis does not evolve in linear fashion. At this point in the report, neither the analyst nor the reader-as-imagined-analyst can know what might come next. And yet this analysis undoubtedly has a history, and Mr. G's observation likely has some kind of status and weight in the analyst's mind. At a minimum, the patient seems to be alerting the analyst to the fact that he is concerned with, thinking about, and has specific beliefs about the analyst's desire. He appears worried that the analyst will be displeased, unsatisfied. (Recall that Racker emphasized the patient's knowledge of the analyst's desire.) The patient is already caught up—to some extent—in the dual relation.

What then unfolds is highly instructive, though complex, and in the end not at all straightforward. The analyst acknowledges the patient's concern about how he might react to the patient's way of speaking. Mr. G agrees, and the issue is dropped. Instead, the patient tells his analyst a story that happened during the break, and he recounts the tale with a kind of elegant verve. The analyst listens and is concerned that he is being recruited into a mini-narcissistic celebration. He believes that Mr. G is pressuring him to join in his enthusiasm, and that he is, as Feldman says, "clearly meant" to "appreciate" and "admire" (789) the patient's eloquence and sensitivity.

In unpacking this clinical moment from the point of view of the desire of the analyst, it is important to notice that *a step is being skipped* in the gap between Mr. G's recitation and the analyst's disclosure of feeling pressured: the analyst is in a state of dissatisfaction; he feels under duress, recruited, and at the same time ignored. As we know from the structure of the dual relation, the analyst cannot feel a specific expectation or pressure from the patient unless he is already *pressuring back*, so to speak. In this case, the pressuring back—the conditions of satisfaction being imposed—is about the way the patient is telling his story.

Let's say, roughly speaking, that the conditions of satisfaction have to do with a "non-manic" way of rendering the story (an authentic calmness and pace to the telling) that implicitly recognizes the otherness of the analyst in such a manner that the analyst does not feel coopted, but instead feels recognized and freer to think and respond. Notice that these feelings of dissatisfaction are not necessarily dynamically unconscious, nor are their proximate causes, because they have to do with relatively accessible conditions the analyst is imposing on the patient. While these conditions of satisfaction are preconscious, they have an uncertain relation to unconscious fantasy.

It turns out that Mr. G was correct to be concerned about the analyst's reaction. Upon hearing the patient's enthusiastic story, the analyst reports:

> When I commented on his manner of speaking and how I was expected to follow, to be involved, and to share the experience with him, he seemed for a moment hurt and offended, but then readily agreed, and said he

had thought at the time about how he would describe this experience to me. His friend Peter and he would share stories this way, but I was more of a problem. (Feldman 2007, 789)

At this point in the report, one senses an unspoken yet mutually experienced mirroring, and a slightly worrisome/contested atmosphere. The analyst is not going along with the patient's "program," and the patient feels hurt. This "not going along" can be, and perhaps in this case is, helpful to the patient (we will consider this issue in a moment). At the same time, Mr. G is not wrong in his concerns: the analyst is, in fact, "more of a problem." The analyst had a set of conditions for listening against which he measured his analysand's story. And yet this crucial element of the interaction is elided in the analyst's description of what follows.

In this regard, Feldman's conclusion is telling:

I was thus induced to feel that I had perhaps behaved in a mean and unsympathetic way, and to doubt the value of the approach I was adopting. ... When my interpretive comment suggested that I was not fitting in with what he desired, I was made aware not only of the sudden eruption of hurt and resentment, but also a vague and ominous threat. (790)

Here, I believe, we have the dual relation/talion law emerging more clearly: the analyst rightly describes his not fitting in with the patient's desire, but he does not recognize that his own desire for a specific experience (which the patient did not satisfy) set the conditions for his countertransference response from the start. (Another analyst may have imposed a different set of conditions on the patient with another result as a consequence.) This is a subtle version of Racker's clashing of desires or paranoid ping-pong.

I describe this interaction as a subtle version because Mr. G does not appear to challenge the analyst directly; instead, after feeling hurt, he is readily agreeable. (In Jessica Benjamin's language, the patient "submits.") If he had been more active and persistent in expressing his concern and hurt to the analyst, then the full brunt of the bidirectional force of the dual relation would be palpable in the room. The patient does not do this. Instead, later in the session and in the following one, he mentions a worrisome mole on his mother's cheek. He associates to a dream in which he

was squeezing or pinching his mother's face, on the cheek where she had the mole. She began to complain, and he saw from her face that she was in pain, and then he became very comforting and reassuring, patting her face, and playing it down as if he had not done anything at all. (2007, 790–1)

Feldman concludes as follows:

> The dream offered a concrete representation of Mr. G's pressure on the object to comply, as a means of denying psychic reality. ... It was clear from the way this material emerged ... that it was also a communication about the eruption of a resentful, hateful attack on the analyst, by whom the patient felt frustrated and injured. (791)

In light of the dual relation and the analyst's desire, it is difficult to know where the "pressure on the object to comply" originates, because both parties are pressuring the other. But this much I think we can fairly say: the patient already understands something about the analyst's desire, and tells this to the analyst at the beginning of the session. But the patient as interpreter of the analyst's experience (Hoffman 1983) is not recognized by the analyst, in the sense that the analyst does not take account of his own desire and the conditions of satisfaction that he has imposed on the patient to begin with. This misrecognition of desire engenders a series of moves by both patient and analyst. Mr. G retaliates for having been hurt. But then he becomes compliant—he submits to the "procedure" underway—avoids challenging the analyst in any sustained manner, and instead produces dreams in which he is hurting his mother/analyst and minimizing the hurt he has caused. In a *mirroring* relation, the patient has identified with the analyst's minimizing of his own hurtful actions in relation to the patient. Without the analyst having a place for his desire in his theory, the understanding of countertransference experience and the parsing of countertransference contributions becomes a difficult, if not impossible, challenge.

My intention in discussing the case of Mr. G in such fine-grained detail is to illustrate the dynamics of the dual relation/talion law in a clinical encounter in which the wider countertransference perspective holds sway. In such a perspective, the analyst's desire is at play and has discernible and at times adverse effects but remains unrecognized and untheorized. And I believe this can have unfortunate clinical consequences. But it is also true that, in order for psychic change to occur, the analyst must often enough specifically position herself in precisely the way Feldman describes himself doing—namely, by refusing to go along with the patient's expectations, and calling attention to those expectations instead.[10]

---

[10] Renik calls this not going along "refusing the [patient's] deal" (1993b, 148).

In the most felicitous circumstances, the analyst, through experiencing the impact of projective identification, shares in the patient's experience so as to differentiate herself from it. However, this differentiation can only be *incomplete* if the analyst does not take her desire as a unit of measure. Sharing can become self-other confusion, and can lead, in turn, to the patient's subtle compliance/identification with the analyst. In such a situation the "analytic object" (Green 1975; Ogden 1994), based on a third position outside the dual relation, is obscured, lost.[11]

To summarize the main points of this section: the dual relation/talion law renders the wider countertransference perspective not only problematic, but also largely unserviceable. The analogical assumption—the "what is going on in me is likely going on in him"—begins to look like a further extension of the basic mirroring structure of the dual relation and an exercise in misrecognition. In this context, the theory of projective identification risks becoming more a rationalization for the analyst's denial of the nature of her own involvement than a clarification of the patient's internal experience. One begins to appreciate that the vectors of force cannot go in only one direction, from patient ("contained") to analyst ("container"). The vectors of force *must* be bidirectional. Finally, the patient may be left in a position of alienation in relation to his analyst and the analysis. Kirshner's (2011) perspective is relevant here:

> Without some form of engagement by the analyst in which his desire is more overtly in play, more transparent, the treatment process is open to covert suggestion, compliance, or an iatrogenic state of confusion or solitude that has little to do with the patient. (4)

## Desire, Responsibility, and Analytic Action

The central focus of Lacan's *Ethics of Psychoanalysis* ([1959–60] 1992) is the question of responsibility for one's desire and, secondarily, for one's actions. The phrase "one's desire" is a composite term that in the *Ethics* means something like who am I in relation to my history? What have I done? What do I want to do? And, what will I possibly do in the future? Each of these questions is problematic and conflictual; they each bring out our eccentric

---

[11] The analytic object, at its base, is loss itself. Loss conditions separation, difference, and representation. We might say, therefore, that the dual relation involves an illusion of plenitude in which loss is lost.

position in relation to our own living. Lacan subsumes all this under the heterogeneous term "one's desire." He puts forward an imperative that is entirely singular and specific to each individual subject, including the analyst. This is the imperative to grapple in an ongoing way with all of these aspects that constitute one's desire.

Some readers may be aware that, late in the text, Lacan makes the following statement that has over time achieved iconic status: "The only thing that one can be found guilty of is giving ground relative to one's desire" (1992, 319). Much ink has been spilled parsing this apparently straightforward sentence. Lacan appears to mean that one ought to go, like Antigone, beyond the pleasure principle, beyond the desire of the big Other (read: normative culture and law), and risk anguish, even exquisite suffering, and a kind of sublime "second death" (Žižek 2007).

I think this is a simplistic and misleading reading. One gets a sense of something more complex when Lacan says, "When an analysis is carried through to its end the subject will encounter the limit in which the problematic of desire is raised" (1992, 300). And a little further Lacan links desire with tragedy and desire's ultimate price: death. The path of desire, in short, is "not a path one can take without paying a price" (323). There is nothing straightforward, then, on this question of desire, action, and guilt. The key point that I take from Lacan's perspective on psychoanalytic ethics is that "not giving ground relative to one's desire" means the *assumption of responsibility* for that desire in all its complexity, in all its "problematic" (Ruti 2012). Guilt (or perhaps more perverse or dissociated solutions) arises for the analyst if she fails to come to terms with her desire, her own actions (including inactions) and her responsibility for them within the treatment situation.

In the context of twenty-first-century psychoanalysis, such a formulation of desire and responsibility, especially as it applies to the analyst and her actions, may appear one-dimensional, and perhaps naive (Kirshner 2012). After all, analysts have spent the last thirty years problematizing unilateral notions that divide analyst from patient. For example, Ogden (1997) does not separate (nor does he think one can separate) transference from countertransference: "I do not conceive of transference and countertransference as separable psychological entities that arise independently of, or in response to one another, but as aspects of a single intersubjective totality" (78). Meaning in psychoanalysis is "negotiated" (Pizer 1992), and resistances are cocreated (Boesky 1990). Analysts contend with an intersubjective analytic field that is sometimes colored by "bastions" (Baranger, Baranger, and Mom 1983) and "retreats" (Steiner 1993). Psychoanalysis is characterized by an interactive "matrix" (Greenberg 1995), and a "relational unconscious" is a core aspect of intersubjectivity and "thirdness" (Gerson 2004).

The concept of the analytic third, in fact, is often thought of as providing a way out of the dual relation by marking a crucial difference between self and other; though, in other hands a more intersubjective emphasis tends to stress that things get shared in analysis. Like Winnicott's transitional object, the third (and its first cousin, the analytic object) is neither the analyst's nor the patient's, and instead is a key part of the field in which the two find themselves. In light of this seemingly overwhelming contemporary picture of analysis as cocreated and shared, it may appear difficult and perhaps misguided to talk of responsibility for one's desire and the actions one takes.

As important as these notions of psychoanalytic practice are—and I believe *the field* and *the third* to be concepts of some significance—they also can lead us to a purely phenomenological view of analysis in which the rough edges are smoothed over, differences are obscured, the inherent asymmetry of the analytic relationship is clouded, and the problem of our own action is, as Lacan says, "masked" by our theory, to return to this chapter's epigraph.

As I described in detail in Chapter 5, my strong preference is to lay stress on the lack that marks each of us as desiring beings, on the fact that we are divided internally, and that our ethical responsibility as analysts is to own the consequences of this basic fact as best we can. The analyst cannot help but instantiate lack, desire, and internal difference in her clinical functioning. Crucially, this instantiation is precisely where the therapeutic power of analysis lies, if the analyst not only accepts reluctantly but also embraces willingly this basic working condition. In such cases it is much more helpful for the analyst to, as Renik says, play her "cards face up" on the table, rather than more or less hide behind a false mask of silence and anonymity. If lacking, then the analyst is open to the effects of her actions, including the possibilities of repair.[12]

Unexpectedly, however, this analytic position I just now described and endorsed goes *against* Lacan's actual clinical stance. Dany Nobus (2016) writes:

> Lacan, much more than Freud, engaged in lengthy reflections upon what he designated as "the position of the psychoanalyst," not only with regard to the aims and objectives (the ethics, the ends) of the psychoanalytic process, but also, and more fundamentally, with reference to the vexed

---

[12] My thoughts in this regard are consistent with what Benjamin (2004) calls the moral third and with Bollas's (1989) dialectics of difference. Benjamin writes that the moral third involves "the essential component principles of the lawfulness involved in repair ... and develops into truthfulness, respect for the other, and faith in the process of recognition" (442).

issue of how psychoanalysts may counter the inevitable impact of the divided subject in themselves. Lacan's proposed solutions to the problem changed over the course of his seminars, yet he *always rejected* the possibility of the psychoanalyst, as agency of the clinical process, operating as a divided subject. (20, emphasis added)

I have spent much time combing through the *Ecrits* and Lacan's various seminars to find places where he states clearly what Nobus describes. I can locate no such statements. Whether such explicit statements can be found or not, I think that Nobus is correct in his assessment.[13] There are moments when Lacan appears to assert the kind of latitude that I am advocating here: "I am always free in the timing and frequency, as well as in the choice of my interventions" ([1958] 2002, 588). But this claim is made within the context of a harsh critique of those analysts who act with their "being," by which Lacan means act with their ego or personality. Further, it turns out that the "choices" Lacan alludes to are fairly limited; from start to nearly finish (that is, until at least 1970), one encounters a view in which Lacan emphasizes the (putative) rigor of the proper analytic position. He writes, "the more [the analyst's] being is involved, the less sure he is of his action" (588). And being sure—or "more" sure—of one's actions is of central importance for Lacan. The analyst, therefore, is described as a cipher, a "dummy" (as in the game of bridge), and often is silent. Through this silence she serves as a cause of the patient's continuing to speak. If the analyst does intervene, she does so always within the terms of the analysand's discourse—the vagaries of this speech, its pace, repetitions, opacities, pregnancies. She does not involve her "being" through the offering of thoughts, feelings, or reveries to the patient.[14]

But the value placed on being "sure" of one's actions is precisely the point of difference I am emphasizing here. Lacan failed to take his assertions about the ontology of the subject—our divided, lacking nature—to their logical conclusions as regards the analyst and her position. The book that you are reading, in its entirety, which is so indebted to Lacanian ideas, runs aground of those ideas on this most basic of issues: "the possibility of the psychoanalyst, as agency of the clinical process, operating as a divided subject." Being is always ineluctably trafficking in non-being, or a want-to-be; this is the heart of the analyst's futural, gyroscopic position. As divided, as lacking and desiring, the analyst's "being sure" is always partial; and rigor,

---

[13] I want to acknowledge a debt to both Dany Nobus and Bruce Fink for their helpful discussions with me about this very issue.
[14] I described in Chapter 6 some of the ways in which Lacan unfortunately brackets the phenomenological, experiential features of analysis.

however comforting, may be hard to distinguish from rigidity, since rigor can take on Imaginary qualities (i.e., the ego's narcissistic features that I described in detail in Chapter 3). The analyst can imagine herself quite secure in her silence, as she toes the line of "rigor" at the expense of a more messy, yet alive and "real," engagement with her patient.

## Clinical Vignette: Byron

Speaking of ethics and responsibility risks sanctimony, and if so, this is a price I am willing to pay for acting on my desire in writing this chapter. In truth, nothing lies beyond my (or anybody's) responsibility, no matter how well-conceived the value upon which the action rests, or how hard-won is the position one has taken. In this light, I want to describe a clinical vignette in which the very analytic value that is the topic of this chapter—responsibility for one's action and the desire that motivates it—itself becomes the immediate source of a dual relation/talion law dynamic. In this vignette, the dual relation resistance lessens once I as the analyst grapple with and take responsibility for the direct impact of my desire on the patient. Then a deeper, more pervasive, and entrenched issue comes into view. This more pervasive issue has to do with my analytic style and usual way of working, based on commonly shared analytic values—in this case, open-minded listening and containment.

Byron, a man in his early forties several years into his analysis, comes into his session upset with his father, with whom he had had a conversation the evening before. This upset leads Byron to revisit several key memories of similar interactions with his father, some dating back to college and his earlier growing-up years. In Byron's eyes, his father is a moderately successful man who rarely shows what Byron calls "backbone." "And he doesn't even know," Byron would say, "what backbone is."

Byron's sentences gather steam as he moves from traumatic memory to traumatic memory, piling on his complaints with avidity. I have heard these complaints many times before. I register internally a sense of disappointment and mild impatience as I listen. I wonder if he is complaining about me. And I wonder what else he might be contending with.

Eventually, I say: "You have a torrent of complaints today about your father. I wonder if the intensity of your feelings is protective somehow, or helpful in your dealing with something more disturbing or scary."

I did not expect to speak in such a carefully disquisitive fashion, and I was surprised at my use of the word "torrent." Immediately, I sense that I have betrayed a feeling of which I had previously been only dimly aware: my seemingly mild impatience was in fact marked and accompanied by annoyance. In the ensuing silence, I do not consider the conditions of satisfaction I am imposing on the patient. Instead, I ponder other possible sources of my annoyance and quickly land on a certain entitlement or implied uniqueness in Byron's recitation of his misery.

My internal musings cease when the patient says: "'Torrent' is a strong word." He is then silent for a minute or two. Feeling a weighty tension between us, I ask him what is on his mind.

"I'm thinking about why did you use that word and how I'm feeling. Why did you say that?"

"Because it was descriptive of how you were speaking," I say with an authoritative tone.

"Maybe so. But you said I was protecting myself."

The weighty silence goes on. Then I say: "Sounded to me like you were protecting yourself. It's a possibility." My sense at this point is that Byron is trying to reach me somehow, but I am still feeling uncomfortable with my "self-division"—that I had said something I had not "intended" to say. I want to rewind the tape, but I can't, so in effect I "double down" with my authoritative tone.

Byron responds: "Well, I was taken aback by the word 'torrent,' and the more I think about it, I think you were protecting yourself, trying to stop me from talking more. That *you* were afraid."

I know, at this point, that he and I are caught in a dual-relation resistance in which attributions are inherently bidirectional (i.e., "you're afraid," "no, it is you who are afraid," etc.). I had not been aware of feeling scared, only annoyed. But it was true that it was I who said the word. Maybe I had been scared?

I say somewhat vaguely: "Yes ... there was something in the way you were talking, an increasing intensity, that I think I was pushing against." At this point I realize that there is no way to figure out who is the fearful party or who started the whole thing; that is a fool's errand. Here, I acknowledge my "pushing." So I ask Byron: "If I were afraid, what do you think of that possibility?"

He replies as if he were laboring against a headwind. "You know, I can go there, and maybe I will, but I still think you want to bypass what happened."

I think, in rapid fashion, about various typical analytic "moves": Byron is turning the tables on me; he's taking over my analytic function; perhaps he's feeling triumphant over me in that moment. These were all ideas that might be true on some abstract level; but in this context they partake of talion-law thinking. Also, these possibilities simply did not feel true because Byron's tone implies a query, even a plea, for me to acknowledge a reality between us, for me to own something that is more mine than his. To interpret any of these putative motivations would simply amount to my retreating from the emotional power of this moment and the responsibility I have for what are indeed mine: the words "torrent" and "protective" and "scary." We are caught in a dual-relation resistance, and it is my responsibility to help us emerge from it.

So I say straightforwardly: "I surprised myself with the word 'torrent,' and just the whole statement generally. I didn't know that I was uncomfortable at that moment, and yeah, maybe scared too. It came out in the words I chose, like 'torrent.'"

At this point, the atmosphere in the room changes somewhat—the analytic atmosphere becomes less contested and fraught, and I feel, instead, open to new possibilities and more curious than anything else as to what might come next. It is close to the end of the session and Byron tells me that he had been worried that I would keep stonewalling him. "I don't know exactly what I'm feeling," he says. "I guess less confused and not so alone."

It was not until a few weeks later that the significance of this session emerged more fully. Byron tells me that he had had a fight with his girlfriend, Susan. During the argument, she had told him to stop yelling and that he was scaring her. She started to cry. Then, to his surprise, he started to cry too. After a while, as they were talking more calmly, he thought of our session from a few weeks prior: "The 'torrent' session," he explains to me. "It came back to me in—well, a torrent. And the word 'torment' came to me, too."

"'Torment?'"

"'Cause I knew I was tormenting Susan—and, I think, scaring you after you said what you'd said. But until you acknowledged feeling uncomfortable, I felt terrible, like I could really terrorize you. It was weirder than that, because I seemed to get what I was doing only after you acknowledged what you were doing. And it made me think about how calmly you listen to me, kind of no matter what I'm saying. On some level I don't buy it, that you're always ready to listen no matter what."

"As if what you're saying is so intense to me that I have to remain calm at all costs?" I ask.

"Yes. 'Cause I can be an asshole. That's what Susan was saying—she was giving me real feedback. And when I said you seemed scared yourself and you clearly thought about that, it was like, 'Finally, he's letting me know he's strong enough to acknowledge the impact I can have on him.'"

I said, "If I'm in my listening, receptive mode, there's something worrisome behind it—that you're so powerful all I can do is take it with a kind of studied calmness."

"I think so," Byron replied. "It's paradoxical. It's the kind of thing my father would never do—tell me what he really thinks."

"When I seem to be strong, for you the fear is that I might really be weak."

"I think so," he said again.

Countertransference is an *activity*: working with one's countertransference does not begin and end with the analyst's desire; it only begins with it. But if the analyst does not begin with it, then the process likely proceeds along the lines of the dual relation in which the analyst confuses her frustrated desire with what is going on in the patient, and the untoward and potentially traumatic aspects of the talion law emerge. In this case the process closes down, the analytic gyroscope is stilled. The general features of this interaction with Byron center on my initial state of dissatisfaction grasped retrospectively, the internal and interpersonal work undertaken in light of the effects of my dissatisfaction, and the somewhat surprising unfolding of his transference experience.

Let us look at some of the details. My using the word "torrent" was a clue to the extent of my unpleasure. I was for a time resistant to my own internal division—resistant, that is, to my desire. What was my dissatisfaction about? Desire gets translated, unwittingly, into unpleasure through terms like *wanting* or *not liking*. We need to translate the unpleasurable experience back into a desire. This kind of translation can sound like clumsy work, perhaps; and yet, when caught in the midst of a countertransference experience, translation of unpleasure into desire can be essential to working through a dual-relation resistance. This translation process gets the analytic gyroscope in motion again.

So here are a series of questions/statements that turn my unpleasure into desire: did I feel tormented by Byron's complaints, as in: I don't want to feel tormented? Did I feel that I was expected to play a certain role in the interaction Byron was fostering, as in: I don't want to play this or that role? Was I reacting in part to the seeming excitement and gratification he was accruing in his complaints, as in: I don't want him to be excited or gratified by complaining? These questions give specific form to my wanting—within the countertransference—one thing to happen, and not another.

I think the third question, regarding excitement and gratification, captures some of what I was experiencing in the countertransference. But this translating exercise is only partially illuminating, because the central problem to which I was responding was, ironically enough, the issue of responsibility itself. To my ear, Byron was externalizing blame and making room for his torment in the comfortable quarters of victimhood. Here I imposed conditions on Byron that he was not satisfying, conditions based on a central value of my working analytic self and one that typically I do not question: Byron was not taking responsibility for his own struggles. Hence my pointed use of the word "torrent."

Byron, to his great credit, pursued this clue in spite of, or more probably because of, my internal struggle to grapple with the desire that underwrote my response to begin with. It was not clear what he was hoping for, and he himself only later discovered that he wanted recognition of the impact on me of his own desire to torment. But without my being able to work internally with my own self-division and lacking state—and, in this case, saying something out loud to him about this state—I believe the rest of the work would not have unfolded as it did.

If I had conceptualized the interaction as Byron having "induced" in me a state of mind (say, that I felt tormented or scared by his complaining), I would have taken myself out of the equation as an actor who necessarily desires. In other words, I would have falsely inhabited an Imaginary place in which judgment regarding my actions—the heart of ethical reflection— does not apply to me. The dual relation/talion law would have become more prominent, and vagaries of bidirectional attributions would have clouded the analytic field, leading to an increasing sense of confusion, upset, and possible trauma. *In the end, the patient is not responsible, from an ethical point of view, for the analyst's actions or states of mind.*

If the analyst does not take refuge in the convenience of considering her experience to be the result of projective identification, then she has gained some purchase on her desire. The analytic process can proceed, therefore, relatively unburdened by the confusion of self and other; the specter of the dual relation/talion law yields to the further emergence of the analysand's voice: his subjectivity, associations, and fantasies. (We might think about this in Winnicottian terms: a "truer" self can come forward now that a "falser" self is less necessary because the analyst has resumed her proper place of lack, and with it the desire and the openness that inhere in that place.) Byron came to grasp experientially not just his desire to torment, but more his desire to see the real impact of his wanting to torment, and that I was "strong" enough to acknowledge this impact, rather than simply receive it calmly, contain it, and name it.

Generally, problems with the analyst's desire emerge when wishes get naturalized within ways of working clinically—that is, when specific desires and values underwrite and inhabit the analyst's clinical theory and actual technical activity (Schafer 1983). When naturalized, a desire or value will then become indistinguishable from the analyst's style and habits of mind, and from what the analyst believes she is rightly doing at the moment. This issue was operative between Byron and me, as my typical listening style that emphasizes my desire to be open-minded and receptive involved me in a cul-de-sac of which I was not aware.

All analysts struggle with their own versions of this problem, which tends to emerge into the clear when the analyst's desire is more open and takes both analyst and patient by surprise (as it did in this case). This dialectic of habit and surprise, I would say—following Lear (2011)—is marked by irony in that the analyst's best intentions, honed from years of training, thought, and experience, will inevitably get in her own way.

No doubt, for most of us, our everyday clinical self partakes of certain basic psychoanalytic values: honesty, tact, open-mindedness, and the like. We might think of these as psychoanalytic virtues. But from the point of view of Lacan's *Ethics* (1992), the virtuous analyst is not one who is temperate or open-minded, tactful, or prudent. Rather, the virtuous analyst takes responsibility for wanting to act in these ways in the first place. Otherwise, tact can ossify into a self-protective caution and open-mindedness can turn into an unthinking and unending receptivity. This is the essence of Lacan's ethics of desire: *nothing should be taken for granted*. In this ethic of responsibility—never not hard-won and always easily lost sight of again— the analyst frees the analytic couple (potentially and relatively speaking, of course) from a dynamic of contest and constraint. If the analyst cannot assume responsibility for her own desire, then there is no way the patient can assume responsibility for his desire, in that setting, with that analyst.

# Conclusion

Roy Schafer (2009) suggests that analysts should catalogue, to themselves, specific ways in which they can become frustrated. That is, what leads a given analyst to be unsatisfied about a specific interaction with a patient? As we know from Klein, the analyst's countertransference arises from states of mind that are particular to a given analyst at a given clinical moment. And yet, haunting the present moment are past moments and larger, deeply rooted concerns that condition our present-tense experience.

Here we can see the value of the analyst's personal analysis: it is the place where she confronts the basic conditions of her subjectivity, and the various reasons (unconscious and conscious) why she wants to be an analyst to begin with. Some of us are highly epistemophilic: we want to understand. In such a case, we tend to feel dissatisfied with uncertainty in all its forms. Others of us wish to be empathic. This leads us to avoid aggressive feelings that we might have toward the patient, and, perhaps, to avoid confrontation for fear of being "mean." Still others of us wish to help and cure, and hence we feel frustrated if the patient does not appear to be aided by an intervention, or does not seem to be improving over a longer-time horizon. And still others among us have fairly explicit views on what constitutes open-mindedness or emotional contact—views that inevitably manifest themselves in conditions of satisfaction we impose on our patients.

Obviously, these are simplistic descriptions of desires that have long personal roots and that interact in most of us in complex ways. Our unconscious need for being loved, desiring excitement, and repairing in fantasy those we feel we have hurt underwrite much of what we experience in more attenuated, conscious forms in the wishes I have just briefly mentioned. But the basic point remains that each of us is motivated by highly personal exigencies that are finely honed into our ways of working, our technique. Our technical activity, no matter how well practiced, thought through, and evolving over time, is never not fueled by our desires. These desires are engaged whenever we experience what psychoanalysts call countertransference.

# 8

# The Ethical Foundation of Analytic Action

*The question that we must continually engage is the nature of our action as analysts. How do we give an account for what we do? What are the parameters that guide us in this effort? We are especially challenged when we find ourselves acting in ways that we can't account for with any certainty. What we bump up against is something hitherto unsymbolized, unthought, and is felt in an action that gets stuck or breaks down. In these moments the analyst fades as subject. My claim is that these experiences of interruption, dislocation, of fading, and our ongoing engagement with them, constitute the heart of the ethics of psychoanalysis.*

*We shall give up the idea that there are special classes of processes that prepare or propel mental activity, that is to say, classes that are qualitatively different from the mental activity they prepare or propel; for now everything is an action.*

—Roy Schafer, *A New Language for Psychoanalysis*

*An ethics essentially consists in a judgment of our action, with the proviso that [the judgment] is only significant if the action implied by it also contains within it, or is supposed to contain, a judgment, even if it is only implicit. The presence of judgment on both sides is essential to the structure.*

—Jacques Lacan, *The Ethics of Psychoanalysis*

After Schafer and Lacan, Renik (1993a, 1993b) and Friedman (1993, 2007), and, more or less, the entire relational tradition (Harris 2011), it is by now a commonplace to say that psychoanalysts are interested in their own activity— that is, our activity, what we are doing with our patients, what we, as analysts, say, feel, and imagine. Analysts have grasped the ways in which their internal worlds shape, illuminate, or constrain engagement with, and perhaps the very emergence of, the patient's subjective experience. The analysand talks in the hope we will receive the other's message generatively, openly, all the while taking the risk that we might misrecognize, not hear, and fail to witness what he wants us to recognize, hear, and witness. This risk involves, as Shulman (2016) says, "a bid for utmost intimacy" (706); the emotional stakes are high. In this context, it is no wonder we care deeply about how we act and why we act as we do. This is why what we concern ourselves with is fundamentally an ethical concern, and why, as Lacan says in the epigraph above, an ethics essentially consists in a judgment of our action.

Importantly, in his *Ethics* seminar Lacan (1959–60) stresses the fundamentally ethical character of Freud's model of the mind as one of conflicting forces or desires.[1] There is a scene, an "other" scene, in which wishes and fears, imagined actions and embodied certainties, get played out, in real time, on the mental stage of psychic reality. As we know, such scenarios tend to emerge within the unfolding drama of the analytic relationship, engaging analyst and patient in an ever-present "happening." The extent to which a human drama is unfolding is the extent to which both patient and analyst find themselves in an ethical field in which each must take account of, and ultimately avow, his or her involvement and impact. Lacan emphasizes, further, that that most basic of Freudian maxims, "Where it was there I shall become" (or, more commonly rendered, "Where id was there ego shall be"), is inherently an ethical exigency related intimately to the becoming of the subject through the process that is psychoanalysis: will I take up that place in which I find my desire, hitherto unknown to me, but now known to me through my experience in analysis? Do I dare disturb my universe? As I described in Chapter 7, this assumption of a desiring position is inherently challenging. Jamieson Webster's definition of desire nicely captures the challenge involved in living as a desiring subject: "Desire ... is a movement that works in and through risk and failure ... [and] bears an intrinsic relation with loss, with the delicate history of one's most intimate and frightening wishes" (2011, 21). The question "What do I do now?" is, then, part of this movement of risk and failure; it is a question we hope every analysand comes to ask him- or herself, increasingly, over the course of

---

[1] Phillip Rieff (1959, 1966) described some of the complexities in the moral underpinnings of Freudian theory, captured in his concept of "psychological man": the monadic modern subject shorn from more authoritative and stable cultural structures. Rieff's work details Freud's role in fostering fundamental changes in Western culture's understanding of what it means to be a person.

an analysis. The patient's "coming to ask" is a possibility dependent on the analyst's capacity to do the same, as I will illustrate below.

Before diving more deeply into these matters of action, judgment, and desire, I want to make two related points explicit. The first is that it is important to distinguish rigorously between *ethics* and *morality*. The fundamental ethical questions are something like: What is the good to which I am aiming? How do I practically go about things? Did I accomplish what I set out to do? Was my action felicitous or infelicitous? What does living well consist in? The fundamental moral questions are something like: what is right and what is wrong? What is it my duty to obey when freely considering a course of action? These latter questions reach beyond a particular person's actions in pursuit of a specific goal and toward a moral law of universal value. And with any value that aspires to the universal—such as mental health, "genital sexuality," or "mature" object-relating—we traffic in an appeal to something all of us ought to be doing or pursuing. Kant's categorical imperative—in which any moral choice based on the use of reason can rightly be said to be the choice that anyone should make—leads, as Bernard Williams has written, to a "morality system" (Chappel 2015). Attempts at establishing a general theory of how one should act cannot help but be, in the end, both pernicious and empty. Williams (1985) writes: "Almost all worthwhile human life lies between the extremes that morality puts before us" (194).[2] There are many reasons Williams was deeply skeptical about the possibility of a foundation for morality or ethical life, but for my purposes the main reason is that the psychoanalyst is always interested in the particular, the singular, the first-person point of view. To make a paradoxical generalization, we psychoanalysts are *anti*-generalists. We know that generalizations about the mind take a back seat to whatever is emerging in the hour as it shapes, *après-coup*, the significance of what has come before, and sculpts, *avant-coup*, the particular as it emerges out of a pluripotent future.

The second point is that judgment of our action is essentially a giving an account of how well the action accomplished what it was consciously intended to accomplish. That's it. It's an assessment that is separable from questions of right and wrong in the sense of obligation or duty. Thus, the analyst sits within an ethical field because our activity is always at play and potentially in question regarding what we are trying to do, why we are trying to do it, and whether we have accomplished what we set out to do. The judgment Lacan has in mind, then, is not a matter of morality, of right and wrong, of one's obligation to conform to some set of external (and

---

[2] See also Lear (2003). For a contrary view, see Annas (1993).

putatively universal) directives.[3] Of significance is the ethical force of a given situation—its conditions of exquisite specificity in which the analyst is called upon to act. The action taken (i.e., what is expressed, done, thought, felt) has direct implications for the analyst's, and the patient's, future commitments (Altieri 1996).[4]

With this as something of an introduction, I want to look at the Lacan quote in more detail and use it to illuminate key aspects of the ethical in psychoanalysis.[5] Here is the quote again: "An ethics essentially consists in a judgment of our action, with the proviso that [the judgment] is only significant if the action implied by it also contains within it, or is supposed to contain, a judgment, even if it is only implicit. The presence of judgment on both sides is essential to the structure."

An ethics involves an action—speaking, let's say, or moving through space—and judgment, or reason.[6] This definition draws our attention to the subjective, embodied aspects of an action. I want something to happen. I have a goal, a telos, and try to make that thing happen. The implicit judgment that Lacan refers to is the reasoning that inheres in the action itself, or is implied by that action; the way, in other words, that I go about bringing off the action. And then there is a second, more explicit judgment: How did it go? Did my action accomplish what I set out to accomplish?

We have two different and interrelated aspects of action defined here: action as the carrier of judgment (or reason) and, on another level, action as the object of judgment.

The latter kind of action—action as the object of judgment—is the essence of science: third-person, seemingly clear, measurable, objective. Here we can

---

[3] We know that some analysts, especially those early in their career, feel constrained and inhibited (if not downright "bad" about themselves) because they are not adhering to an imagined set of ideals of "analysis" from which they find themselves forever straying. Also, all analysts, at times, can veer into moralizing territory, especially when we feel under threat (see Goldberg 2007).

[4] Schafer (1976, 1983) demarcated much of what I am discussing here with his seminal, brilliant, and (unfortunately) mostly forgotten work on "action language." Schafer's effort was to move psychoanalytic theorizing from reification of abstract concepts (e.g., instincts, defenses, states of mind, and locations such as inside/outside) to language more appropriate to human experience-as-activity, to the language, that is, of action. However, while innovative in the extreme, Schafer did not frame his work within the larger field of an ethics of psychoanalysis, let alone investigate its territory in depth.

[5] Other significant writers on ethics in psychoanalysis include Chetrit-Vatine (2014) (see this book's Chapter 2), and Kristeva (2014). They emphasize a central aspect of ethics that I do not discuss in any detail here: this is the "matricial" care or responsibility for the other (e.g., child, person, patient) that redounds to the analyst because of the asymmetry—and hence the emotionally powerful nature—of the analytic relationship.

[6] As some readers may recognize, Lacan's definition is essentially that found in Aristotle (see the *Nicomachean Ethics*).

report the degree to which a given action succeeded or failed, describe its ongoing effects, and the like.

The former kind of action—action as the carrier of judgment—ends up being phenomenologically complex, resolutely first-person, and difficult to capture in symbolic terms. We are, in other words, decentered subjects often motivated by unrecognized desires to which we have no privileged access; we get only a glimpse of our desire in retrospect, through what we do or, more importantly, through what we try yet fail to do. In the "failure" of a consciously intended action (e.g., a slip of the tongue) we experience a dislocation, a fading of self, as this misstep seems to arise from some other place in us. What we bump up against is something hitherto unsymbolized, unthought, and is felt in an action that gets stuck, interrupted, that breaks down. My claim in this chapter is that these experiences of interruption, dislocation, of fading, and our ongoing engagement with them, constitute the heart of the ethics of psychoanalysis.

There is a further subtlety here that requires emphasis: the "both sides" that Lacan refers to applies not only to two aspects of judgment of our action, but also to both sides of the analytic dyad. In the end, if unrecognized desire and experiences of dislocation are the heart of the ethics of psychoanalysis, they are no less so for the analysand than for the analyst. Both analyst and patient come to take account of their implicit judgments, unknown desires, and enigmatic actions through the process that is psychoanalysis.

## Action as the Object of Judgment: Ultimate Aims and Ends of Analysis

First I want to look more closely at the second aspect of Lacan's definition: action as the object of judgment. The "How did it go? Did I accomplish what I set out to accomplish?" Such questions have broad applicability, from moment-to-moment interactions within a given clinical hour all the way to the end of an analysis, the broad sweep of its results, its outcome. Namely, did the analysis make a difference, and, if it did, what kind of difference did it make?

In fact, there is significant debate within the field whether to consider psychoanalysis a treatment procedure at all, which would make assessment of our reasons for action as analysts potentially more mysterious, both to us and more especially to our patients. For Renik (2003), the goals of analysis must be clear, and directly related to the patient's suffering, namely, his symptoms and their alleviation: "Failure to keep track of therapeutic benefit and to make technical choices on the basis of whether symptom relief is being achieved leaves an analyst wide open to dangerous complacency about his or her work. It spares the analyst accountability at the patient's expense" (36). For Purcell (2014), the psychoanalytic task is distinctly *not* about a therapeutic treatment: "Psychoanalysis conceived and conducted as a set of techniques used to deliver a 'treatment' must be out of touch with something integral to the [patient]'s experience of emotional distress" (800). Lear (2009) has written about the same set of issues regarding the goal of analysis, what he calls its "final cause": "Freedom is the final cause of psychoanalysis: freedom is the kind of health that psychoanalysis aims to facilitate ... freedom of mind, freedom of speech and freedom to be and let be—all of which can be considered as aspects of freedom" (309–10).

While Renik uses phrases like "technical choices" and "symptom relief," Purcell argues that routine application of "a set of techniques" runs counter to being in "touch," to making meaningful contact with the patient's "emotional distress," and so would tend to contribute to further distress. The difference between these two points of view represents a tension that runs deep within the field, and in the heart of any analyst, and might be captured in the following question: How do I use a generalizable technique in a personal way, a way of being an analyst that shapes itself to the requirements of this particular patient? Renik (2003) writes:

> Customarily in psychoanalytic circles we speak reverentially of case-specific factors, of the uniqueness of the clinical moment, and we look with great skepticism upon generalizations that might threaten to efface the complexity of these particulars. "It depends on the individual" might well be a motto emblazoned on the psychoanalytic coat of arms. There are many colleagues for whom technique is in itself a dirty word because it is understood to denote a rigid code of behavior that would make them insensitive to their patient's individuality. And yet we realize that responsible clinical practice requires us to think about what we are doing and to develop, if possible, principles that we can apply across cases and across moments to guide ourselves toward optimal patient care. (50)

Lear's perspective is more overarching and subsumes the concerns of Renik and Purcell. After all, a final cause or ultimate aim is for the sake of which all other efforts are made (e.g., contact with emotional distress, amelioration of symptoms).

There is no beating around the bush about the fact that our field is more than a little confused about this crucial issue of ultimate analytic aims.

In spite of this confusion, my intention here is not to wade more deeply into these "ends-of-analysis questions," and what the ultimate aim of analysis ought to be. Instead I want to emphasize that these questions are fundamentally ethical, because they relate intimately to judgments of our action and, by implication, to our responsibility (or as Renik says, "accountability") for our action as analysts. Judgment and responsibility go hand in hand: to consider seriously why I did something and how it succeeded or failed, I would have to, at least implicitly, take responsibility for that action. This accounting is, without question, an activity that one can reasonably expect any psychoanalyst to be able to do.

## Action as the Object of Judgment: The Now-and-the-Next

I want to turn from the very broad question of the ultimate aim, or final cause, of analysis, to the opposite end of the spectrum: the moment-to-moment interactions in the now-and-the-next of the clinical hour. I am still in the "How did it go?" or "How is it going?" aspect of judgment of our action: Is the analytic process going well or not? As a way into this issue, consider the following scenario, one that made an impression on me years ago as a candidate, and one that many analysts have experienced: this is when we, as a candidate or trainee, present clinical process to a supervisor. These moments are so common as to go unnoticed, perhaps. Consider the moment when the supervisor, as we are reading our process notes, is, to our dismay, shaking his head in disapproval. He does not like what he is hearing. Or, on the other hand and to our great relief, we look up from our notes and see him nodding his head in assent. This time he likes what he is hearing. What is happening in these moments? Our supervisor is imposing *conditions of satisfaction* on the work. Often our supervisor is well versed in how he assesses the quality of a clinical hour, and what conditions he is using (imposing) to make that assessment. What is sometimes strange about our experience with our approving or disapproving supervisor is that he may have a hard time explaining what he likes or doesn't like about the given interaction being described. That is, the standards by which he is measuring the clinical work are less than sharply formulated in his mind. He knows a good analytic process when he hears it, as well as what he considers to be "not analysis" at all, but this is often by feel, as he struggles to lay out exactly what conditions he is imposing on the process in order to assess it. This is a struggle that all of us deal with in some measure, and the extent to which we impose conditions of satisfaction on our clinical work but can't account for what those conditions are is a measure of an ethical failure on our part because the very capacity for judgment of our action, and the possibility of taking responsibility for that action, are noticeably incomplete.

We face the same set of concerns as analysts with our patients. As I described in detail in Chapter 7, it is a rock-bottom fact that we are imposing conditions of satisfaction on patients (and ourselves) all the time—inevitably, unavoidably, necessarily. This imposition is how the psychoanalyst has a chance to make a meaningful difference. A more down-home way to say this is that we want certain things to happen and not others. For starters we want patients to show up for their appointments. (Though we would "roll" with a no-show and take up that issue with the patient next time.) We want them to speak to us once they arrive. (Though silence is, at times, a necessary state as well.) We want them to listen to themselves as they speak and to listen to us as we speak to them. And we ourselves want to be open-minded, curious, and imaginative about what the patient is saying and not saying. If they don't do some of these things we call it "resistance." And if we don't do some of these other things we call it the "analyst's resistance," or "countertransference." What is crucial here is that the analyst's desire—what the analyst wants to have happen—conditions the field, establishes a certain standard for work, and is the foundational base without which what we call countertransference would not exist. These conditions are usually implicit, and often unconscious. It is one of the marked ironies of psychoanalytic work that we are responsible for what often enough we are unaware of or take for granted, or when we act in ways we didn't expect or can't account for. To the extent we can catch hold of it at all, the desire that inheres in our action comes to us in retrospect, after the fact. And our responsibility for our desire is double. We both acknowledge to ourselves (and sometimes to the patient) the conditions we have imposed, the action we have taken. We also, and more importantly, listen for its impact on the patient and the process.

## Action as a Carrier of Judgment, or Reasoning-in-Action

What I have been describing thus far is the explicit judgment question, the "How did it go?" question, whether from the point of view of the ends-of-analysis or the moment-to-moment interactions of a given hour. And how the entire analytic landscape so mapped—from its vast topography to its smallest features—is ethical in nature. Second, a constitutive element in all of it is the desire of the analyst, what I have called the "conditions of satisfaction" the analyst cannot help but impose on the patient, on herself, and on the process.

Now I want to move onto the harder-to-grasp part of Lacan's definition of an ethics essentially consisting in a judgment of our action—this is the implicit judgment aspect, the "reasoning" that inheres in the action itself. If I am thirsty, and I start walking toward Death Valley in search of water, we could rightly say that the action I am taking is inherently unreasonable; this unreasonableness is independent of whether I might luckily stumble upon an oasis in Death Valley. If I am a psychoanalyst, and my job is to listen to the patient, it would be unreasonable to use earplugs to accomplish that task, even if, in the end, the patient appears to change in positive ways.

The basic set of conditions that we inhabit by deciding to be analysts implicates us in an unusual circumstance. We know that any interaction in which we are involved can become, all at once, the immediate topic at hand. But how can we anticipate such moments? We can't. They come into view in the approaching horizon of the next. This is an important reason why these moments have ethical force: they call us—interpellate us—to give an account of what has happened and is happening; to fully implicate ourselves in this unfolding actuality by speaking to it in the here and now, and remain as open as is possible to what happens after that.

By simply considering the unusual circumstances I have briefly described here, we can appreciate that within the reasoning that inheres in a given action in psychoanalysis there will always remain a gap between what we think we are doing in that moment and the account we give of it after the fact. It is commonly understood that an analyst's self-description of what she is doing and why is often at odds with others' perceptions of what she was doing in a particular case. We implicitly perform meaningfully to our patients in ways that often belie what we are explicitly saying or doing. As a result, we deceive ourselves if we think it is a straightforward matter to offer an account of what we want to have happen in a given clinical moment or what in fact is happening in that moment. It's one thing to look back over the broad sweep of an analysis, itself an enormously complex task; it's quite another to give a compelling account of something happening in the now-and-the-next.

Jay Greenberg (2015) approaches this issue of reasoning-in-action from the point of view of the incommensurability of competing psychoanalytic theories and how they might account for a specific clinical moment in an analysis. Greenberg uses a case vignette described by Civitarese (2005)— in which a patient, during the final session before a holiday break, pleads for Civitarese's advice about a family crisis—and examines it from different theoretical perspectives. Each different perspective Greenberg calls the analyst's "controlling fiction." He argues that there is no way to adjudicate which perspective deserves to be endorsed or, on the other hand, dismissed. This epistemological puzzle aside, Greenberg's larger point is an ethical one, as he tightly links the analyst's theory, or "fiction," with his responsibility to act. Confronted with a felt challenge that requires a response of some kind, Greenberg says: "The analyst, faced with the need to choose quickly among a multitude of available responses ... filters the possibilities through a theory of therapeutic action" (2015, 28). While the analyst participates in the unfolding action, he also, as Greenberg emphasizes, must make "clinical choices" (28); each "fiction" leads to something quite real, as the analyst's working theory, in some measure, obligates the analyst to act in a manner consistent with it.

The picture Greenberg paints—from the point of view of the individual psychoanalyst in the trenches who is challenged to act—lacks a certain experiential and conceptual precision. Greenberg confuses the first-person with the third-person point of view. This is because the analyst in the trenches, at that exigent moment, is not considering her options to act and the reasons that underwrite them from the point of view of a "fiction." The analyst has a particular view of therapeutic action, based on beliefs about the mind, human relationships, and the purpose of psychoanalysis for the patient lying before her, a view that she believes has a basis in fact. This belief does not imply certainty, or any other rigidity. Further, this lack of certainty (an inherent condition of being an analyst) does not suggest that the analyst acts on the basis of what she considers a false belief, that is, on the basis of a fiction. The analyst believes what she believes to be true.[7]

I have suggested how difficult it is to connect truly avowed reasons for action with the action itself and whatever reasoning might be carried within or through the action. There will always be a gap between avowed reasons for action, the action itself, and our retrospective reading of what happened. (This is made more complex, of course, by the interpersonal nature of the analytic situation, influenced not only by the impact of the analyst's desires but also by the patient's various demands and wishes.) For example, here are my avowed reasons for action given the situation Civitarese describes: I would act, or attempt to, with a sense of my ethical responsibility for the other (Chetrit-Vatine 2014), motivated by a desire to maintain the analytic relationship and the continuity of the analytic work. I would try to keep sharply in mind that my position is necessarily partial, lacking, conflicted. Regarding what

---

[7] As the literary critic Stanley Fish writes: "If one believes what one believes, then one believes that what one believes is *true*, and conversely, one believes that what one doesn't believe is not true" (1980, 361, italics in original).

I might say to the patient, I would reference the dilemma she faces especially in light of the upcoming break, modulating my words to address or at least indicate her affective state and sense of urgency. Depending on her response, I might get further into the details of the crisis she feels she is facing. But, whatever the specifics—which obviously cannot be described in advance—I say what I say and do what I do "knowing" that I can't possibly know what I am doing, both in the doing and in what will come next. I find myself acting as much as I choose the action, and usually more so, especially in moments of emotional urgency. And what follows, what emerges in the next, in the futural and anticipatory moment of the patient's response, is most significant (Schlesinger 1995; Faimberg 1996, 1997). In this light, what does "reasoning-in-action" look like? Can we even assert its existence, if the analyst is finding herself acting as much as, or more, than faithfully carrying out something planned? I can only agree when Altieri (1996) observes, "our most passionate actions tend to reveal far more than the performing consciousness takes account of" (82).

Regarding Greenberg's "guiding fictions," only from the abstracted, third-person point of view, in which the imagined perspective is capacious enough to take in the larger psychoanalytic landscape, can one be in a position to see the impossibility of adjudicating the relative merits of each clinical theory. This larger perspective is of a different order entirely than that from which any one psychoanalyst works.

Here, I believe, is the heart of the matter regarding action as a carrier of judgment. It is no doubt true that the analyst, often enough, thinks and plans, feels and reflects, and then may or may not do something other than continue to listen. Even if nothing is "done," the analyst's listening position is changed as a result; or, perhaps better, within and through the process of feeling and reflecting, the analyst is in a different listening position, for the moment. But even in this most usual of circumstances, in which the analyst "thinks and plans, feels and reflects," there is always a place of dislocation. There is no coherent "reason-in-action" in psychoanalysis because there is always, structurally, a difference between "I" and "me," conscious intention and performative message, all informed by unconscious elements of conflict, worry, personal style, and character (Kite 2008). Taken together, these features of analytic action entirely preclude the possibility of self-sufficiency, of self-presence. As Jane Kite writes in her already classic paper, "The Analyst as Person" (2016): "We find ourselves as *individuals* ontologically unfathomable" (1154; emphasis in original). This is a structural fact that conditions a dialectical movement, in time, from here to there, from action to reflection and back, made ethically meaningful by the patient's presence, suffering, and desire for recognition.

## Countertransference Enactment and the Fading of the Subject

If the entire analytic enterprise is ethical in nature, the center of this ethics project, the navel of this ethics—to invoke a telling image from Freud (1900, 111 n. 1)—is in those moments of action in the now-and-the-next in which, effectively, the analyst is inhabiting this gap, deaf to her own desire at the moment, unaware of aspects of the impact she is having on the patient. There is an important sense in which the analyst is always only half-hearing. The analyst believes she is listening, but finds out she has only been listening in a particular mode, and so has not been listening in other modes (Grossman 1999). More broadly speaking, the analyst believes she is being an analyst as she goes about her work—implicitly enacting a way of being that houses within it specific analytic desires and values—only to find through some bit of internal or interactional experience that what she thought she was doing she was not. She was doing something else, and it was having an impact on the patient she did not consciously intend. In short, the implicit judgment that inheres in the action at that moment was off, faulty. At this point the analyst goes about the effort at retrospection I mentioned earlier: What just happened? What am I wanting in this moment, and doing in this moment in the service of this wanting, that has led to this?

We know what to call these experiences, and especially within the contemporary Freudian tradition we have a now well-established literature on this topic. It is called countertransference enactment. Here was the American psychoanalyst, previously under the sway of the autonomous ego, rationality, and deliberation, catching hold of clinical moments of significance "after the fact," after having done things or said things that were not at all expected but could not be denied. It was at this moment that an ethics of psychoanalysis, at least within the American Psychoanalytic Association, was born. These analysts (e.g., Jacobs 1986; Chused 1991; McLaughlin 1991; Renik 1993a, 1993b) wrote very much from within the clinical trenches and with an ethic of candor. Forget, they say, what analytic technique tells us to do; let's look instead at what we actually find ourselves doing. Further, let's look at what we find ourselves doing that our theory does not prescribe, privilege, or endorse, and that our conscious intentions can't explain. It's pretty on-the-ground stuff—pragmatic, useful, and, as I said before, candid. One could write a history of psychoanalysis that traces all the ways in which what once was proscribed as "not analytic" has become a daily part of our lives as psychoanalysts.

But we cannot rest too comfortably at this moment of the "countertransference enactment" and its ethic of candor. We know as psychoanalysts that candor, or a commitment to telling the truth, is never a straightforward affair, for at least two reasons: (1) Human desire is variegated and multiple; to affirm one aspect of things is, necessarily, to obscure other aspects. (2) Truth is always in close proximity to lying, just as a negation is a way to acknowledge something as true while claiming it is not.

Certainly the earlier work on enactments opened up an ethical field in which, often enough, our activity is frankly acknowledged as ahead of, or out front of, rational deliberation. But I wish to emphasize that the enactment, as a kind of psychoanalytic event, is only the most famous instance within clinical psychoanalysis that demonstrates its fundamentally ethical character. In fact, I would argue that the loudness of "enactments" obscures, and even distracts us from, this fundamentally ethical character of our work.[8] Here I am getting back to what I alluded to earlier: the heart of the matter when talking of an analytic ethics, its center, with reference to Freud's metaphor of the navel and the unknown.

Consider a recent clinical moment in which the analyst is caught up short: perhaps it was the tone of voice we used in speaking to a patient; or a break in the frame, such as inadvertently ending a session early. Or maybe it was something we usually take for granted, like the look of our office or our style of dress. Or even such unassailable analytic values as open-minded, nonjudgmental listening. But this particular time the patient makes an issue of it: as in, "Don't you have any opinions or reactions to what I am saying?" The list of such moments, of course, is nearly endless. These moments point to something previously unthought and unimagined, something suddenly real, like a pebble in one's shoe or a chicken bone caught in one's throat—something that demands attending to, taking stock of, speaking about. Humphrey Morris (2016) describes these moments in analysis as "living the real," moments the analyst struggles to acknowledge and tends to disavow defensively.

If we think about how such moments feel, we can appreciate that they capture something essential about the basic working conditions of being

---

[8] Boundary violations (i.e., sexual or other exploitation of the transference relationship) involve the moral dimension of psychotherapeutic work, as opposed to the ethical field I am describing in this chapter. Boundary violations are, obviously, outside the limits of any responsible professional practice. They are, in a word, bad or wrong, and we designate them as such. This explicit proscription emphasizes how important it is for any analyst to respect that limit of intimacy and passion that we all bump up against, but that must be approached, if necessary, for the analysis to make a significant emotional difference.

an analyst. These analytic moments of living the real have a particular phenomenological quality: it feels as if we have momentarily vacated present experience only to be brought back to it as we grapple with what has just happened. We were "somewhere else" for that brief period of time; this "somewhere else" we experience as a kind of forgetting or absenting of our self. We fade as subject, and then we "come back." "What was that?" we ask ourselves. "What just happened?" "What did I just do, or the patient and I just do, and why?" Or "Yes, I can see that I was taking something for granted that is now very important, very present between us."

This fading and coming back points to a dialectic of self-experience in the analyst that circles around a gap or lack; this lack is constitutive of what it means to work as an analyst and goes far beyond the famous example of the enactment. There is an important sense in which the entire analytic endeavor involves this fading and coming back that continually shows itself to us in a way that we experience as a kind of forgetting or absenting. And this is why I harked back to Freud's classic image of the dream's navel, its "point of contact with the unknown" (1900, 111 n. 1). The ethic of candor so admirably foregrounded by those who wrote about enactments takes on, within the basic working conditions of the analyst I have outlined here, a paradoxical cast: we find ourselves, or refind ourselves, where we thought we had been but had not.[9]

If the id, or the it, is the unthought, the unrepresented, the unknown, then Freud's ethical maxim where *it was there I shall become* applies not only to the patient but, more importantly for our purposes, to ourselves. As psychoanalysts, in moments of forgetting, of fading, we must then take up that absent place so as to be poised in a futural, anticipatory attitude open to what emerges next. If we refuse this lack, this absenting, then the opportunities for the patient to respond and speak are blocked, foreclosed. But they are blocked only until we come back to this absent place, in which the psychoanalytic dialogue has a chance to get going again. Most crucially, if the analyst struggles with the fact of her own dislocation, and elides her ethical responsibility for this otherness within, then the patient will be left alone, alienated not only from the analyst but also from his own desire and the shadows of its insistent presence. In such a case there is nothing for the patient to avow, and no possibility of asking crucial questions.

---

[9] This chapter is about the ethics of the analyst's action as analyst. But, as I have alluded to in several places, I don't mean to suggest that the same set of ethical conditions do not apply to the patient. In the end, they do (though we might debate the different kinds of responsibility that redound to analyst and patient).

## To Close, for Now

I would like to circle round and close with a story about the ends of analysis, the broad sweep of an analysis, and the analyst's contending, in real time, with the "How did it go?" question. I was a candidate and my supervisor was Joseph Weiss. I was having problems with exactly the "How did it go?" question, what amounted to my reluctance to take responsibility with how things had gone. The patient, a talented but traumatized and sad young man, had made significant and lasting changes through our work together. In the final weeks of the analysis he was struggling to find ways to express his gratitude for my having helped him. One day in supervision Joe says to me:

> "Tell him that he feels very lucky to have met you. That's what he's been trying to tell you. Can't you see that? How fortunate he feels to have stumbled into your office five years ago."
>
> "I can't tell him that," I say, almost pleading. "That's way too much, way too much tooting my own horn."
>
> "Bullshit," Joe says. "You tell him that because it's the part of the truth he can't say, and he can't say it unless you let him know you can hear it."

# 9

# The Proleptic Unconscious and the Exemplary Moment in Psychoanalysis

*In light of what I have offered in the foregoing chapters—the enduring voice, the otherness of speech and the matricial, the forgings of closure that mark the ego, desire and lack, the ethics of countertransference and analytic action—with all of this, a question remains: what is the nature of the unconscious?*

*Prolepsis (pl. prolepses; pron. prō-'lep-sēz):*
*anticipation, such as*
*a: the representation or assumption of a future act or development as if presently existing or accomplished*
*b: the application of an adjective to a noun in anticipation of the result of the action of the verb (as in "while yon slow oxen turn the furrowed plain")*
—Merriam-Webster Dictionary

*Life isn't about finding yourself, or finding anything. Life is about creating yourself, and creating things.*
—Bob Dylan, *Rolling Thunder Review* (Film, Martin Scorsese)

I want to talk about a central and mostly overlooked aspect of the unconscious as manifested in the clinical work of psychoanalysis. This is its proleptic nature. The unconscious is proleptic in that it performs futural possibilities for the subject. These futural possibilities emerge as potentially significant in the now-and-the-next of the analytic hour—that is, immediately (all of a sudden), or later, whether later in the hour or in further times to come. Manifestations of the proleptic unconscious, moreover, effectively anticipate objections from the past self that is now called into question by the emergence of the potentially significant. In the "character neuroses," for example, the formal repetition of obligatory ways of seeing the world and one's relations within it—the patient's "past self"—may struggle with its very transformation into a somewhat altered position; in other words, the analysand and at times the analyst may "object" as he or she moves into a future that now presents different possibilities than were previously imagined or known.

I have used the phrase "the-now-and-the-next" rather than the "here and now" throughout this book because the former phrase captures better the futural position we all live in, including when working as psychoanalysts. I borrow from Heidegger the picture of human being as being-in-the-world, in a certain mood that conditions experience, and in anticipation of the not-yet. We are thrown into the world, are practically engaged, and so care in a naturally forward-leaning, anticipatory manner. Heidegger's term for this being-in-the-world is *Dasein*, which he defines as "that entity which in its Being has this very Being as an *issue* for it" (1962, 32, emphasis in original). The most obviously repetitive phenomena that we observe in psychoanalytic work are always before us within the moving moment of the present into a future sculpted by the horizon of death in the distance. In this sense, what is repeated is never the same; it is never the identical iteration over and over. Even if, phenomenologically speaking, the repetition feels deadly, static, oneric, it is never only that.[1] And even if the analyst intervenes precisely about this deadness—the "emptiness of the repetition"—what is most important is the next thing that happens: how the patient responds, what comes up next for the analyst in her associations, and the like. As McWilliams writes (sounding Heideggerian): psychoanalytic therapy "has a self-righting mechanism that iterates toward authenticity" (2004, 42). The analyst, then, is a caretaker of the treatment in the Heideggerian sense: she leans into the future open to what is realized in the next, ready to mark it, attend to it, just as she is simultaneously marked and attended to by it.[2]

This ongoing participation in life as necessarily anticipatory does not mean such participation is free from projection. Heidegger's picture of *Dasein* is embodied participation in the doing of life and so involves the person in a futural, leaning-forward position that does not rely on cognitivist

---

[1] This is a point that Oldoini (2019) makes quite powerfully in her recent paper on traumatic development.
[2] One would not want to make a fetish of the immediate moment; the dialectic of *après-coup* makes the immediate inherently Janus-faced, as it points simultaneously toward the future while potentially reconfiguring the past. Laplanche's model of the spiral is helpful in conceptualizing this double movement (1999, 231).

assumptions such as prior beliefs or desires. In this picture, projection is, let us say, empty and open to new possibility within the ongoingness of acting and living. Contrast this, for example, with Lacan's mirror stage, which is all about the human being projecting—anticipating—a better self, a more together, ideal self, in a futural space; a projection that is false and thereby constrains, even deadens, what lies before the subject ([1949] 2002, 75–81). This is just one well-known example of how one might limit, through projection, future possibilities. The analyst works against this narcissistic trend in herself, works against this tendency to fill the emptiness of the next with a picture of it, especially a picture of how the analyst wishes to see herself in that next moment (or wishes the patient to be in that moment). The analyst's position is gyroscopic: moving and therefore decentered; lacking and hence informed by a well-honed analytic desire.

The proleptic unconscious shows itself in a turning or pivoting—a changing of direction, like a crossover dribble in basketball. Intimately related to the analyst's position as "gyroscopic," the proleptic unconscious is a becoming, as a kind of arrival or the entering of a new place. But the challenge of representing this turning or becoming is considerable. We are all of us tempted to concretize and reify. In what follows, I argue against a view of the psychoanalytic unconscious as having a locale or space that is content-filled. I will spend some time giving shape to what is in the end a formal moment, since the psychoanalytic unconscious as conceived in this chapter—what I am calling the proleptic unconscious—is without content. It is the "to be realized." My emphasis throughout will be on the performative function of psychoanalytic actions. I use the plural "actions" to include those found in the clinical examples I will soon describe, the performative role of the clinical example itself, and the possible impact on the reader of this very writing (including the possibility of its utter failure to impact the reader).

I start with a discussion of the performative role of the clinical example, as this idea sets up what follows in the rest of the chapter. I offer three detailed vignettes that attempt to capture a central feature of the proleptic unconscious, that formal moment of turning or becoming. In the middle section I spend time highlighting ways in which analysts emerging out of the ego-psychology tradition struggled with the problem of reification of the Freudian unconscious. These analysts, such as Grossman and Simon, Loewald, Schafer, and Renik, among others, attempted to move beyond the stumbling-block of reification by emphasizing ways in which representation of unconscious contents or functions are, in an irreducible way, dependent on the language of human desire (wanting, needing, fearing, and the like). This dependency establishes the terms of the manifestations, or better, realizations of the unconscious within a human field of acting toward future possibility and emerging ways of being, as contrasted with the persistent expression of the extant, repetitive, and always already known (a reified unconscious). These analytic writers anticipated the proleptic unconscious.[3]

## Exemplary Moments and the Futural

It is not unusual in psychoanalysis for the clinical example to be denigrated as merely one instance among any number of others; clinical examples pile up as so many untested hypotheses.[4] Yet, in psychoanalysis, as in the arts, any given instance can extend, through its performative impact, beyond the single case it describes. In his paper, "Example and Exemplification," literary scholar Charles Altieri makes this point persuasively: "Example allows the particular itself to have scope: Hamlet becomes a type because of what he does, not because he instantiates some principle" (2015, 130). We might say, following Altieri, that Hamlet "happened," or better, "is happening": Hamlet sees his father's ghost; he feigns madness; he mercilessly scolds his mother in her bedroom; he foregoes opportunities to murder Claudius.

When a literary example takes on scope and becomes a type, it serves an exemplary function. Altieri (2015) again:

> Exemplification is oriented toward action rather than the simple recognition of underlying conditions. And exemplification points toward future uses rather than ideas of capturing some abiding core of wisdom. It is we who adapt the test to the world by showing it helps us sort experiences and specify how they matter as means of determining values. (131)

We don't think of Hamlet as instantiating principles or categories such as hallucination (the ghost) or Oedipal disgust (the merciless scolding). Instead,

---

[3] This chapter was originally written for the *International Journal of Psychoanalysis* North American Centenary, in Rye, New York, October 2018. This occasion, including especially its locale, stimulated me to focus on American psychoanalysis; hence my emphasis on some of the central contributors to this particular topic from the United States. In addition to the analysts I discuss here, other important writings on the problem of reification and time have come from Lacan (1981), Faimberg (2005), Roussillon (2011), Parsons (2014), Civitarese (2016), and Stern (2018), among others.

[4] As is well known, from the point of view of mainstream scientific method, any single case report is, at best, hypothesis-generating; only by other methods can hypotheses be tested for their validity.

we imagine these actions—that is, we place Hamlet in a setting doing these things—and use such staged moments to help us sort and understand present experience, just as we might use a clinical vignette we have heard about or read or experienced ourselves to assist us in engaging an analysand in real time, in the now-and-the-next of the work.

The everyday travail of analysis rarely, if ever, find its way into our clinical literature. Micro-moments of a given analytic session may well be involving for the analyst as she attends to subtleties of interaction, dialogue, and atmosphere. An extended silence can be riveting. Yet, reporting these subtleties in a vignette is likely to put the reader to sleep (if in fact there is a reader to begin with). A botanist may be fascinated watching grass grow, but such a rate of change is far too slow to hold anyone else's interest. From an outsider's perspective, an actual psychoanalysis is almost unfathomable, so prosaic, so every day, is the work (working through, after all, can take years). At the same time, this very "everydayness" is a necessary condition for anything meaningful to happen in an analysis.[5]

From the point of view of the everyday, psychoanalytic clinical writing is a different species from psychoanalytic clinical practice. The clinical moments typically reported in the literature are decidedly not of the everyday variety. Again typically, the moments described attempt to capture a rapid rate of change—immediate, often dramatic, and usually of great emotional and cognitive significance. Often, perhaps nearly always, the analyst is a central character in the story that is told; she is a character of epic endurance ("making the best of a bad job") and canny sleuthing, as the hitherto obscure becomes the finally revealed (Wilson 2016; Mulligan 2017). Not only must one hold the reader's attention, but also as writers of psychoanalytic literature we hope to capture in the rendering of endurance and revelation exemplary moments with which the reader identifies, takes as significant, and gives value to. While we don't know with certainty that such exemplary moments are truly as therapeutic as is often claimed, they do serve a meaningful rhetorical (i.e., persuasive) purpose: that something important happened—is observed, experienced, described—and that the analyst's desire to analyze is momentarily fulfilled. Regarding the patient's experience in the analysis, clinical moments of potential significance become so as they are emotionally and cognitively impactful. A few such moments may rise to the level and take on features of the exemplary, an experience that is often shared with the analyst; but whether shared or not, it is so subjective that the analyst may not fully appreciate (or even know) that such an event has transpired for the

---

[5] For some patients, the analyst's care, commitment, and the resolve such work entails may be both necessary and sufficient conditions for therapeutic benefit to accrue.

patient. Here I am referring not only to the "logic of unveiling" (Baxter 2008) one commonly finds in the psychoanalytic vignette, but also to those patients for whom something that the analyst said or did had enduring impact, while the analyst was the last to know (Renik 2006).

Regarding psychoanalytic writing, such a moment qua clinical example has a chance to become more than a single instance; it may itself become exemplary. At such times, the stark difference between analytic work and analytic writing dissolves.

Arguably, *the* exemplary moment in psychoanalytic literature is not from the clinic; it comes from Freud's observations of his toddler grandson playing. The Fort! Da! story serves the function of the exemplary in precisely the way Altieri describes: this single moment less proves an underlying principle or condition—how could a single example "prove" anything?—and more serves as an example against which we can "test" future moments, help us "sort" them so as to invest them, or not, with value. Each of us might perform this testing in a somewhat different manner, using different terms. For me, the Fort! Da! story allows the sorting of clinical moments around questions regarding a patient's capacities for the representation of absence (i.e., the absent and potentially traumatic object), his or her openness to play and relative tolerance of separation and difference. The Fort! Da! serves this exemplary function by allowing me to relate present experience to Freud's grandson's use of a pair of phonemes, a piece of string and a toy train, playing the game of "gone" and "there" as his mother is absent. Here I explicitly place emphasis on a specific psychoanalytic value, namely, the importance of the capacity to mediate sense experience and to represent—and thereby contain and think about—loss, broadly speaking.[6]

This example from Freud is about the analyst's use of the exemplary in working as an analyst. The patient, too, as I have already suggested, is open to the possibility of the exemplary. When such an exemplary moment happens in an analysis, the patient is impactfully interpolated into futural possibilities that had up to that point been inchoate, resisted, only partially engaged or considered. These moments intervene proleptically ("point toward the future") as much as reflect the already known (an "abiding core of wisdom"). This pointing toward is an opening for something more, the "not-yet." At times, possibility entails relinquishing, and this relinquishing can be no easy task for either patient or analyst. The patient wishes, in part, to reaffirm the present state of affairs, and the analyst, also, in her own fashion,

---

[6] The absence of this capacity (so-called unrepresented mental states) falls within the orbit of the question of representation about which the Fort! Da! orients us.

has a tendency to repeat basic principles and tenets and ways of being as if continually answering a deep concern about the very foundations of working psychoanalytically.

Kravis makes this observation about clinical writing:

> It might be fair to say that some analyses take a very long time because it takes the analyst a long time to become that patient's analyst. The best clinical writing should reflect this process of becoming. Every working clinical analyst is a latent memoirist. (2017, 800)

And somewhat later in the paper: "Clinical writing ... separates itself from self-display and the ethos of hypertransparency insofar as it aims to depict precisely such acts of becoming on the part of the analyst" (805).

Kravis's emphasis on "acts of becoming" is entirely apposite regarding necessary transformations in the analyst over the course of an analysis (an issue I will take up in Clinical Example 3, below). As I have been describing in the early pages of this chapter, this is also true of the patient. Such "acts of becoming" are precisely the manifestations of the proleptic unconscious that are my focus here. Such moments can be described, written up, and shared with colleagues in the hope that they work in precisely the futural and exemplary way Altieri describes in the quotation above.

## Clinical Example 1: A Turning from Nothing to Something

Molly stood in front of her bedroom mirror with a silver letter opener in her hand. It was mid-morning. Her husband was already at work, her sons at school. She angled her chin to the right and surveyed the left side of her neck. She had always admired her fair, pale skin. This time she noticed scars from previous attempts. One near the bottom of her ear. Another under her chin. These did not deter her. This time she would make the punctures count. And regarding time, it was of no moment. Or rather there were no moments, only the present, her face in the mirror, her neck exposed, letter opener in hand. Like a gull in a steady glide over the shore at high tide, Molly lingered over her neck, looking, surveying.

Momentarily, she put the silver opener down on the dresser. Resuming her gaze in the mirror, she took two fingers and pressed them into that space on her neck where she could feel the pulse of the carotid artery. It took a few seconds and, as she searched for her pulse, she noticed something on her left hand. On a fleshy finger of that hand. Her red nail polish was chipped off. And there was her wedding ring. A bevel-set diamond, in need of refurbishing. This ring, to Molly, at that moment, was a surprise, or an intrusion, an interruption. Though at that point nothing much changed. She continued her search for her pulse. The ring continued to intrude. Soon thereafter she had a thought about the ring, as if the ring had a thought about her: "You are married." "Oh yes. I remember now. I am a wife." And then: "You are a mother." "Yes, I am a mother."

Molly called her husband and told him she needed to go to the hospital; he came home and brought her there. She told me this story upon discharge, ten days later, when I took over her care.

To put things perhaps too simply, Molly was saved by the bell of the symbol, the ringing of signification. It was fairly accidental. If she had had more interest in the other side of her neck and used her right hand to check her pulse, the moment might never have happened. This happenstance was part of Molly's engagement with her wedding ring. She had been lost in a fugue, forgetting who she was, where she was, and with whom she was. She was instead enamored by, in a way in love with, the search for that exact place she would puncture her skin with the opener. As near as she could get to the carotid.

And then—it took a few seconds—Molly's split-off removal (what we tend to term dissociation) shifted, as if clicked off. She then knew who she was, where she was, and with whom she was. Later, when relating this story to me, Molly said she was "shocked into" finding herself back to reality, and to know, at the same time, that she had been completely mad only moments before. *A ring became her ring.*

We can certainly say that prior to the wedding-ring moment Molly was not conscious of her status as a subject—that she was a wife, mother, professional person, and the like. This entire world was foreclosed to her. Then these features of her self—the "objects that one is to oneself," as George Herbert Mead (1934, 136–7) said of the nature of the self—became visible to her. Molly's place in her particular world was now locatable: "I am here, in this place, and I live here with my husband and sons." She "sheltered her responsibility"[7] through the mediation her ring-as-signifier provided her. The immediacy of her capture by her own mesmerizing image was broken. She became human again in that moment. And it is important to notice how Molly's experience of turning from nothing to something falls within the scope of the Fort! Da! example: she finds a way, or a way finds her, to represent her experience and herself in that moment. Like Freud's grandson

---

[7] This felicitous phrase is from Lacan (1993, 188).

and his toy and his phonemes, Molly, with her ring, finds her place, however precarious her hold on that place might be.

The example of Molly illustrates one feature of the proleptic unconscious, or at least a key aspect of its manifestation—that it emerges as a turning or pivoting within a temporal flow, in a form (from punctate to extendedly elaborated) that disrupts conscious attention. One's sense of reality, and one's place within that reality, twists, at times rather abruptly—a shift in experience based on a shift in attention. I am not speaking of something strictly internal, a psychic reality filled with belief and propositional content. Here it is not a question of the warded off being disclosed so much as a self-state being transformed, on the spot, into something else. In other words, I am not engaging the question of a deterministic psychodynamics, in which an extant set of conflicts must inevitably find expression; and in Molly's case whether her status as subject was split off or repressed or something else. I don't have an explanation for how she moved from state A to state B, except that her ring intervened and rather contingently at that.

Like Freud's story of the Fort! Da!, this moment when Molly gazes at her neck in the mirror and sees her wedding ring is extra-clinical. She and I had yet to begin working together. It was a key aspect of the story she told me of the circumstances that led to her being hospitalized. Later, in a four-times-per-week analysis (conducted vis-à-vis), all manner of associations and conflict about her status as a woman, her struggles with each of her parents (including deep and enduring identifications with a psychotic and home-bound mother)—all of this "past" history emerged in the now-and-the-next of the clinical work.

This kind of painstaking effort is, for most analysts, the essence of psychoanalytic treatment—the gradual elaboration of a history, in part the repressed, forgotten, dissociated, or simply minimized history, of the development of a symptom or a structure of psychopathology. This elaboration, of course, evolves and shows itself within the dynamic unfolding of the analytic relationship. Even with this more conventional psychoanalytic work in which a painful and traumatic past is brought into the treatment relationship, worked on and partially worked through in the present—even here, the proleptic unconscious is alive, as Molly revisits her past and in so doing moves into a future of more possibility. As I have said, the proleptic unconscious interpolates the subject into the future. It is, in this sense, fundamentally the realization of the new.[8]

---

[8] Even the transference is, as Poland (1992) described, an "original creation." Also, note that analytic work with the "unrepresented" or the "absent" in highly traumatized patients involves the *ongoing creation* of a substrate of affectively meaningful words,

## The Freudian Unconscious and the Problem of Reification

Perhaps the reader might justifiably believe that I am artificially splitting past and future, repetition and prolepsis, enduring content and emerging process. If so, I am doing it to highlight the latter terms in these binaries, terms that tend to get short shrift if not ignored altogether. Difficulties present themselves both theoretically and clinically if the futural nature of the proleptic unconscious goes unrecognized, and if, on the other hand, the psychoanalytic unconscious is viewed primarily as a space filled with extant content that is organized deterministically. The central conundrum is how to intervene in the futural direction I have emphasized, in a way that has a chance to lead to something new and potentially valuable, when the object of interest—the psychoanalytic unconscious—is always already there? This dilemma is especially puzzling to think through if we impute content to this unconscious, whether it be fantasy and wishes, object relations (which involve fantasy and wish), anxieties and defenses, and the like. The most anodyne results are obtained, as we end up where we began, finding exactly what we were looking for. Renik puts the problem this way:

> Nor is it easy to adjudicate on empirical grounds the validity of different expectations that cause us to infer, or not to infer, the existence of unconscious thought, since the observations we use to make our evaluations are themselves always strongly influenced by the very expectations we want to evaluate. (2000, 5)

In short, the rabbit is never magically pulled, de novo, out of the analyst's top hat.

In spite of these very real cautions, without question the kind of careful work I briefly alluded to in the example of Molly is central to psychoanalytic clinical investigation. If there exists a foundational principle upon which all of psychoanalysis rests, it is the psychological impact of the past on present experience, and the belief that meaningful engagement with one's past as it affects the present is basic to psychoanalytic work. This foundational principle or belief is itself based on an explicit or implicit attribution of enduring, extant mental content—"the unconscious"—that must persist in

phrases, and interactional experiences in the now-and-the-next of the present and future clinical hours.

the mind in order for the past to have the effects on present experience that it is said to have. In 1917, for example, Freud writes, "phantasies possess psychical as contrasted with material reality ...; in the world of the neuroses it is psychical reality which is the decisive kind" (1916–17, 368). Phantasies, Freud continues, derive, ultimately, from "primal phantasies ... [which] are a phylogenetic endowment" (369). Thus, the unconscious content that constitutes psychical reality is pictured as an entity, an ontic "thing in the mind" that is atemporal and knows of no contradiction. An unconscious wish, for example, is always pressing for expression and is, qua wish, impervious to any constraints. Countervailing forces do, of course, exert constraints, resulting in a compromise formation. Thus, in refracted form this pressing-wish conditions conscious experience (including the transference); it gives shape to cognitive content and invests it with the tone and hue of specific affects, as Arlow described (1969).

The same basic picture of an enduring psychic reality pertains to the more recent (but still decades-old) emphasis on qualities of mental functioning; that is, the patient's capacities to symbolize, tolerate affect, integrate psyche and soma, distinguish fantasy from reality, and the like. If the patient's mind "works" in characteristic ways, then a key analytic goal is to help him or her see how their mind does what it does regarding these functions. Obviously, if such workings were transparent to the subject, no psychoanalytic attention to this area would be necessary. These workings, then, both endure—that is, they have a course of development from past into the present—and are, at least partially, descriptively and perhaps dynamically unconscious. The ego psychological emphasis on unconscious ego defensive operations is one example of this focus on mental functioning, itself part of a larger attempt to forge out of psychoanalytic theory a "general psychology."

## Anticipations of the Proleptic Unconscious in American Psychoanalysis

My emphasizing the futural foundation of the proleptic unconscious struggles to cohere with this more classical Freudian picture. How can the psychoanalytic unconscious have a proleptic dimension when its two essential features—atemporality and no "no"—stipulate that it is always already there? If the proleptic unconscious is oriented toward "future uses," what about "underlying principles," and an "abiding core of wisdom"? This is not simply a conceptual conundrum generated by the terms I have set up in this chapter. It is one that psychoanalysts, beginning with Freud, have continually confronted. The basic assertion that the stuff of the unconscious is ever-present and affirmative in its seeking of satisfaction seems true and accords with clinical experience. And yet, it also encourages reification of unconscious content of whatever type. As a general matter, models tend to be static; lives tend to be lived.

In looking into these conceptual problems, and their practical consequences, I will lean heavily on writing by Freud, Schafer, Grossman and Simon, Loewald, and Renik, all of whom in their contributions, in various ways, anticipated the concept of the proleptic unconscious. What I believe is fairly easy to demonstrate is that psychoanalytic theorists, especially from the ego psychological tradition in the United States, gradually moved from a picture of the unconscious as reified—filled with stuff always already there—and pressing for expression, to a focus on action and doing, to a mind unfolding and creating in its real-time expression. Specifically, these writers grabbed hold of the question of representation of the unconscious via figurative language, and gradually turned our orientation from the past and the things in it toward the future and the actions that make that future manifest. A more synchronic, structural picture of the mind is replaced by a diachronic one, as mind is now conceptualized as action "in time." Prediction and the expectation of the same via synchronic structure become anticipation through action, a diachronic unfolding, an openness to the new.[9]

The effort to substantify and concretize the unconscious (and the mental apparatus more generally) with the tools of language and figuration has been recognized as a worrisome concern since the early days of psychoanalytic theory-building. For example, in *Beyond the Pleasure Principle* Freud tells us that,

> We should not feel greatly disturbed in judging our speculation upon the life and death instincts by the fact that so many bewildering and obscure processes occur in it—such as one instinct being driven out by another or an instinct turning from the ego to an object, and so on. This is merely due to our being obliged to operate with the scientific terms, that is to say with the figurative language, peculiar to psychology (or, more precisely, to depth psychology). (1920, 60)

Arguably, Freud's "our being obliged" is more accurately stated as "our being unable to do without," which, in turn, leaves us to wonder about the validity of this very distinction between instincts (also forces, tensions, compulsions) and the language used to give such things visibility. What, specifically, is the

---

[9] The metaphorics of this effort are abundant and reach far beyond past/future: binding/unbinding; law/desire; paternal/maternal; dead/live; discovered/created.

"figurative language peculiar to psychology"? One can feel Freud's being caught in the thicket of language as he struggles to be free of it.[10]

Grossman and Simon (1969), in a masterful paper, "Anthropomorphism—Motive, Meaning, and Causality in Psychoanalytic Theory," describe in detail Freud's grappling with this problem of representation of forces and dynamics in the mind. They also powerfully critique the effort by earlier ego psychologists (Hartmann, Kris, and Lowenstein 1946; Hartmann 1965) to render the dynamics of mind in nonmetaphorical, depersonified language. Hartmann, Kris, and Lowenstein substitute the language of "tension" and "quantity" (so-called depersonified terms) for that of "wish," "intention," and "quality" (so-called anthropomorphic language). Whether the effort was Freud's or these mid-century theorists', Grossman and Simon cannily conclude: "Abstract terms which have been substituted for language of intention have ... no other definition than the terms of intentionality for which they are supposed to substitute" (1969, 93).

And later in their paper:

> It is not necessary to "purge" the clinical theory of anthropomorphic language. Anthropomorphic language is in no way incompatible with systematic study of individual cases, or of groups of cases, or with any number of ways of grouping and organizing clinical observations. Anthropomorphism per se is not "unscientific." It serves a number of useful purposes, including that of inviting empathic participation by the analyst. Its value lies in providing process terms for explanation according to motives. So long as the only processes of which we speak are wishing, intending, and needing, and their defensive counterparts, there is no other language available. (107)[11]

Thus, the "figurative language peculiar to psychology" is the language of dramatic action and the human motives that underwrite such action. One can feel in this quoted excerpt movement toward something futural, as the passage is filled with present participles (e.g., inviting, providing, wishing, intending, needing, etc.). We also notice that Grossman and Simon prefigure Altieri with their emphasis on use and purpose, as well as "inviting empathic participation" through the valuing (or not) of the clinical example.

---

[10] For an exemplary instance of literary scholarship on this very question, see Neil Hertz's "Freud and the Sandman" (1979).
[11] As René Rousillion has said: "What we need in psychoanalysis is a metapsychology of process rather than a metapsychology of content" (quoted from Howard Levine, personal communication).

The "action language" of Roy Schafer significantly extended this critique of reification of the unconscious. In truth, an examination of Schafer's groundbreaking work would merit an entire chapter. For my purposes here, the central point to emphasize is that Schafer wished to situate psychoanalytic experience, including models of mind and representations of the unconscious, strictly in the field of human desiring and human acting, in time and embedded within a describable psychological and interpersonal context. He effected this change in orientation through attention to a grammar of motives that better captures the teleology of human action, including the workings of mind in real time. "When speaking of any aspect of psychological activity or action," Schafer writes, "we shall no longer refer to location, movement, direction, sheer quantity, and the like, for these terms are suitable only for thing-like entities" (1976, 10).

Loewald adumbrated Schafer's emphasis on action by asserting, as is well known, that a key aspect of superego functioning is anticipatory. He writes that the superego is "a non-fulfillment of the inner image of ourselves, of the internal ideal we have not reached, of the future in us that we have failed" (1980, 274). Here Loewald captures the role of a motivating internal desire ("the inner image of ourselves") that gives meaningful shape to future striving.

Less well known, perhaps, is what Loewald searchingly offers in the next paragraph of that paper:

> The greater or lesser distances from the ego core—the degrees of internalization of which I spoke—perhaps are best understood as temporal in nature, as relations between an inner present and an inner future. Such structuralization obviously is not spatial. Physical structures are in space and organized by spatial relations. It may be that we can advance our understanding of what we mean when we speak of psychic structures if we consider the possibility of their mode of organization as a temporal one, even though we do not as yet understand the nature of such organization. (274)

Loewald's picture of the relations of structures in the mind as "temporal in nature" is, as he himself admits, hard to see with any clarity, but the suggestion that mind is infused with temporality is certainly offered in a similar spirit as Schafer's more developed ideas on the mind-as-action.

Finally, with the advent of the "enactment turn" in American psychoanalysis in the late 1980s and early 1990s, the question of representation of the unconscious moved from explicitly symbolic tools—the language of human desire—to unwitting actions on the part of the analyst, actions that come to be partially understood retrospectively. In the spirit of Schafer and Loewald, Freud's basic distinction between "remembering" and "repeating" was called into question, as thinking was now seen as a kind of acting. Renik, for example, writes:

> I think we have maintained, without realizing it, what is really an unsubstantiated theory that fantasy can become conscious without having been expressed at all in action. ... On the contrary, there is every reason to conceptualize thought and action on a continuum, thought being a form of trial action, based on a highly attenuated form of motor activity. (1993b, 137)

In the end, of course, the "figurative language peculiar to psychology" remains indispensable; a theory of enactments simply holds that meaning always comes later in the sequence of events in order to give legibility and signification, *après-coup*, to the unwitting and unconsciously motivated actions that enactments are said to entail.

If, as Ricoeur (1977) astutely put it, force and meaning are the two irreducible pillars of psychoanalytic theorizing, then what this effort that I have here summarized amounts to is to argue that force in and of itself *is* meaning; or better stated, that the language of desire makes force human and so situates the subject within the drama of a life unfolding in time, including, importantly, its tragic dimension (Schafer 2007). As I have said earlier in this chapter, the risk to the psychoanalyst in subscribing to the belief that the psychoanalytic unconscious is thing-like, ever-present, and locatable in space is that the analyst will, in the end, simply end up finding what she is looking for, because the extant content is there for the analyst to discover and decipher—activities that are perhaps satisfying to the analyst, but potentially deadening for the analysis.

My solution to the reification problem is to empty the unconscious of timeless content pressing for expression. Instead, it is precisely in time, in the now-and-the-next of the clinical hour, that manifestations of the unconscious are realized or emerge as the potentially significant. It is much less the case that the psychoanalyst "speaks" to the patient's unconscious, and much more so that the patient's "unconscious" speaks to both parties through its proleptic dimension of becoming as the analytic work moves into the future.[12]

---

[12] At this juncture I want to pay tribute to Bruce Reis, whose work I only recently came across. Apposite of this discussion, he writes: "Meanings are not performed, or formed only inside the individual. ... There is no place that meaning is—meaning is a constant

## Clinical Example 2: From Something to Nothing

I have four doors that patients must negotiate as they come and go from a session. Usually this is done without incident. There is the door from the walkway to the waiting room. It is unlocked, and there is no combination. It presents no practical problems. There are two solid-core doors—"double doors"—that separate the waiting room from my office. Each of these doors has a spring-loaded door-drop that engages upon closing, thereby assuring the absolute minimum transmission of sound from office to waiting room and vice versa. These can present problems in fully closing each of the doors; some force is required. Some patients, as they come into my office, choose to close the waiting-room-side door, while I close the office-side door. Other patients simply walk into my office and I close both doors, the second one with my shoulder as I lean in to engage the latch fully into the strike plate. Finally, there is an exit door from my office to the walkway through which the patient leaves at the end of the session.

Luna is an academic, middle-aged, who came to see me some years ago for what she called "a block in my writing." She was having terrible trouble finishing her second book. Luna cut a regal bearing. She had striking features, wore silk scarves, and had noticeably excellent posture, such that I found myself standing a little more upright as I greeted her in the waiting room and perhaps again at the end of sessions as I opened the door for her to leave.

Luna cared about these doors. All of them. Her father had been a carpenter. She knew about latches, locks, strike plates, hinges, and door-drops. About the double doors, she always wanted to shut both of them. She was unusual in this regard, but not unique among patients I have had in my practice.

Not surprisingly, her conscious concerns about her scholarly efforts involved a particular fear: "That," as she often put it, "I will leave myself open to data I haven't considered, or if I have I will have missed its full implications for my research. And then I'm vulnerable to all sorts of counterarguments and criticisms." With this worry a constant threat, everything appeared potentially significant to her, as if she might at any moment miss, or misread, or perhaps ignore the very thing that would inoculate her research and her book project from devastation.

Analytic work with Luna was difficult. She struggled with obsessional worrying that was at times tinged with overt paranoid ideation. I had to be careful regarding my position in relation to her consciously expressed fear that I knew what was in her mind, and a less conscious worry that I could

process of becoming and transforming…. The emergent properties of these truths and phantasies are the function of the enactive field … which is in constant flux" (2010, 701).

intrude into that protected place at my whim. Sometimes she sat up; at other times she used the couch. Her robust internal protections were jealously guarded, lest unwanted thoughts and feelings intrude and wreak havoc. And yet, there was a sense, over time, that something important was being established between us that provided her with a modicum of calm, and her vigilance diminished.

The symptom that brought her to treatment waxed and waned. The thematic nexus of doors and blockages, what she allowed in and what she kept out, her idealization of her father shielding her from moments of trauma and at feeling overwhelmed at his hands—this territory we crossed and crisscrossed many times, in an effort at "working through." Yet, often the work felt labored and heavy, burdened by a seriousness that seemed to signify that more analytic work needed to be done. "Let's keep going," I told myself. Sluggishly, in stops and starts, her attempts at further research and writing yielded some results. But not as much as she had hoped, as she was twice denied promotions. The possibility of something genuinely new happening felt quite remote.

One day Luna "forgets" to close the office-side door as she comes in for her session. We have been working together for about six years at this point. While I can't be entirely sure that this has never happened before, certainly it is a rare event. I note it to her, as I often do regarding nuances and subtleties in her comings and goings.

"I'm in a rush today," Luna explains. "I'd like to get back to my writing. I'd rather not be here. But I'm worried, as usual, about the quality of my work product. So, in that sense I'm glad I am here, to take a break."

The heaviness and tension in the room is palpable, a feeling that is familiar. I choose not to engage the topic of her writing, which can seem, often enough, as if each word spoken is literally adding a gram or two of weight to the room, to the burden that Luna and I then must bear. In such moments an uttered sentence has unwelcome gravity; paragraphs can add up to several kilograms of burden.

After an extended silence I say: "You left the door open today. For me to close it, I think. For me, I imagine, to participate in your life in some way that is physical and constructive. It's a simple thing, for you to want me to close the door behind you, and welcome you in."

"That's true. It is a simple thing. Nothing like finishing my book, which you can't help me with."

I think to myself (as I sometimes do with Luna) that I should tell her a joke, to lighten the mood. But nothing comes to mind. I think about telling her that brief train of thought, but I don't. I also do not believe it helpful for me to "interpret" what some might hear as an "attack" on me as an analyst in her comment "which you can't help me with." This would likely embark us on the divergent path of the dual-relation resistance.

That night, Luna has a dream, which she tells me about the next day.

In my dream is an infant, a little baby girl who is about 7 months old. Something like that. She has never spoken a full word in her life, just baby talk. She's laying on her back, semi-swaddled. I don't really recognize her, though she is of a darker complexion, like me. All of a sudden she says her very first words, perfectly enunciated: "Shut the door, Roberta."

In telling me this dream and especially quoting the young child, Luna laughs freely, deeply. She finds this moment incredibly funny. I am not sure why she does, exactly, though I do notice my body is more relaxed and there is a smile across my face. I somehow get it. Her associations go here and there: "Maybe Roberta is an old neighborhood friend Robert, who I had a crush on when I was 16? He was adorable." She goes on for a minute or two about Robert. Then she is quiet. "Or," Luna picks up again, "I think of my old girlfriend, Rosie, who always left cabinets and doors half open? That was so annoying." She then tells me of fantasies she's had about the double doors in my office and the excellent soundproofing: "It's so well soundproofed that it makes me think that at some prior date you had a problem with it, like somebody in the waiting room could hear what was going on in here. Maybe you were sued?"

"And devastated."

"Well, you're still here. So maybe not."

"But if doors aren't shut real tight someone could get into big trouble."

"That's how I've always felt. Better safe than sorry. I don't want to be sorry. But it's no way to live a life."

"No, it's not."

There is a poignant wistfulness between us that feels important, as we sit in silence for a time.

As the hour is drawing to a close she repeats the phrase again: "Shut the door, Roberta," and chuckles. The wistful feeling has gone. "Sorry," she says uncharacteristically, "but it's so absurd." "Absurd." "Yes. Ridiculous." Luna's laughing to herself. "Those words are nonsense. As my daughter might say: 'They don't mean jack shit.'" She gets up to leave, she shrugs her shoulders and says with a big laugh: "Shut the door, Roberta."

Luna went to her office and worked on the final chapter of her book.

What evolved over time is that "Shut the door, Roberta" came to signify—between us, in the analysis: "Whatever. I don't really know. And I don't have to worry about every little thing. What counts, what doesn't, what is in and what is out. Not everything has to mean something." Luna found this idea (a meaning in itself, obviously) liberating and helpful. Her seriousness lifted some. She was able to write with more freedom from the devastating concern that there were fatal flaws in her work.

As with Molly, Luna had a conscious experience that altered her sense of herself in relation to her world. With Molly, nothing had meaning prior to her moment with her wedding ring. With Luna, everything had meaning, and so she was constrained by a kind of overreading, overinterpreting. Her dream led her to consider that not everything has to be something, that not everything is meaningful. This experience brought her back to the living, rather than being frozen in obsessional worry and paranoid fear. The possibility that some things might be meaningful and others not was an idea that would have made no difference to her if we had talked about it in generalities, as a matter of abstract principle. Luna's dream, its unbidden nature, its experiential immediacy, and the wit of its message—that she found it so genuinely funny—all of this together had impactful significance as she was interpolated into futural possibilities that had up to that point been inchoate, resisted, only partially engaged or considered.

In my estimation, whatever transference meanings one might infer from Luna's dream (and our exchange) take a back seat to its proleptic dimension. Certainly, other analysts might have felt an exigent need to interpret Luna's putative hostility, or her apparent feelings of manic triumph over me as she laughs, telling me (as "Roberta") to shut the door after she leaves my office. From what source, or sources, would such an interpretation issue? Some privileged place from which the analyst summons knowledge or insight? What place is this, exactly? From her countertransference? From a metapsychological theory regarding the human mind? From (in my view) an unwarranted technical principle that privileges "transference interpretation" above other forms of analytic engagement? And why would the analyst invoke such a theory, or give precedence to a feeling, urge, or thought that arrives in herself in such a moment as I encountered with Luna?

My way of working is, as a general matter, to respect the patient's text—in this case Luna's dream—the patient's interpretation of it, and more generally the patient's inherent capacity for growth, rather than impose on the patient an interpretive grid from without. I am interested in helping her as she engages new possibility with the greater freedom she has found; such engagements will likely include further conflict, both in her outside life and within the analytic relationship.

## Clinical Example 3: From Private Citizen to Psychoanalyst

While we cannot help but report from an irreducible distance the workings of other minds (as I have in my descriptions of Molly and Luna), the analyst's self-account partakes of an immediacy that is not possible when discussing another person's experience. But the relative availability of self-experience (feelings, fantasies, inferences) should not be confused with transparency, obviously. As analysts, we will likely find we had been feeling something or stuck somewhere subjectively important only after we find ourselves in a different place psychologically and emotionally. In this final clinical example, I report a dream that interpolates me proleptically as I experience a transformation in myself-as-analyst in relation to myself-as-citizen, a transformation that signified and allowed for a more open and capacious position in relation to myself as I worked with my patient, Thomas.

Thomas is a successful professional in a field in which his judgment and actions are often under attack. He is something of a "born-again" Christian—not evangelical, he is quick to point out. "I'm refinding," he tells me, "my Catholic upbringing." Though this "refinding" has been a long time coming. Thomas's religious training, mostly driven by his mother's passionate involvement with the Church, was observant of Catholic tradition: Sunday school, ritual practices during Lent, Confirmation, and the like. But as he grew into his teens and early adulthood, Thomas felt increasingly distant from the world of the Church. For much of his adult life he viewed himself as an "agnostic," rarely stepping foot into a house of worship. During the past five years or so he has resumed going to church on Sundays, including participating in the Communion rite.

Thomas is also a highly trained firearms expert, and owns many different kinds of guns and other weapons. He holds views on a variety of political and social topics, and is especially ardent about Israel's right to exist free from threat. He sees himself as a "political centrist," and has well-worked out ideas and arguments about the ways in which "political correctness" has compromised, as he often has put it, "healthy political debate." He told me that he voted for Barack Obama in the 2012 US presidential election.

Thomas came to see me some years ago because his wife complained of his irritability and remoteness. He told me he himself had for many years felt alienated from people, at a remove, and lived with an "emptiness inside," although his feeling of emptiness was somewhat relieved when he attended church and participated in ritual. He explicitly registered a closeness he felt when in church to the spirit of his now deceased mother, whom, in his recollections of his childhood, he described as loving and supportive—not idealized, and certainly not narcissistic or overtly traumatizing. It was Thomas's father, a successful research scientist, who was described as distant and self-involved, and who, in his remoteness, was repeatedly hurtful to Thomas.

And it was his father on whom Thomas laid blame for his wariness of other people and his quickness to judge them harshly. Endowed with a keen intelligence and a vigorous work ethic, Thomas excelled even if he at times subtly disrespected teachers and kept a distance from potential mentors. He noticed, and at times worried about, not being interested in other people, feeling unimpressed by them, often harboring negative judgments of them. His views on social and political matters were no help in this regard, as he felt he lived in a community that was "seeped" in a "liberal" point of view.

My approach to Thomas and his struggles was superficially no different than with any other patient: I was curious and interested in his endeavors, whether it be his marriage and children, his job, his political perspectives, or his deep involvement with firearms and questions of safety. I learned much about all of these domains of Thomas's life. He worried that I felt "repulsed" by him, that I was offended by his intensely pro-Zionist stance: "At best, you just tolerate me," he said. There was also—and at times this was made explicit— a worrisome, if fleeting, feeling in the room. I knew, because Thomas told me, that he had canvassed my office for "weapons" the first time he entered it. This is "automatic" for him: wherever he goes, he assesses his surroundings for exits, and scans for objects that can be used, if necessary, for purposes of self-defense.

I told Thomas many times during our working together that his struggles were not only due to an enduringly fearful, even terrified part of himself; they were also, at least in so far as he wished to protect his loved ones from harm, out of his feelings of connectedness to them. He wasn't, in other words, simply and only an empty person who was alienated, removed, and at times terrified. "It is true," he would say. "I'd do anything for my wife and kids." We also spent many hours discussing his feelings of extreme vulnerability and mistrust, linking them to his early history and to interactional moments between us in which he was sure that I "couldn't stand" being with him. My overall goal for Thomas was to help him become more familiar with the parts of himself he hated or felt were completely exposed and unprotected. I also, as I said, pointed out the particular ways in which he went about loving those he was close to.

My conscious transference to Thomas was, in retrospect and in a way that I will describe in a moment, perhaps too unconflicted. I did often ask myself, as he would wonder about my feelings of repulsion for him, if I did at all feel repulsed? Or did I feel afraid? What about his, from my personal perspective, rather brutal view of the Palestinian people and their right to self-determination? As his analyst I was open to all possibilities and curious about whatever he was talking about or struggling with. As a citizen, I was perhaps less charitable toward him. I was, also, less aware of these possible feelings and dispositions until I had the following dream:

> I am in the West Bank, looking for kitchen appliances. That is the "reason" why I am there, though there are no appliances to be found. Instead, I am in a concrete, modest building, with white walls, a bare cement floor with little if any furniture. I am loosely part of a tourist group; we are white, a mix of Jews and Christians, and pro-Israel. But something ominous is afoot. There are "Palestinian terrorists" in military garb with assault rifles over their shoulders standing outside and in a doorway. We're in potential danger, and I try to warn the people I am with that we have to leave immediately: "We have to get out of here! Now! Let's go!" The scene becomes more focused and my visual field narrows as I or we run out of the building. It now seems safe, but quickly I realize it is not. So I run more, and implore others to keep running, or keep escaping. Then things change: I am driving a small car on an overpass, speeding to get out of the West Bank. Now I have a choice to make. I either veer left and head back to the West Bank and face what seems to be certain death, or veer right and make it to safety in Jerusalem. Since I don't know the roads and this decision is upon me all at once, I fear I will turn left and be in danger again. But I lean to the right, nudge the steering wheel in that direction, and know I will make it to safety. Then I wake up.

There are an infinite number of ways that the analyst, through the course of an analysis, changes, is transformed, finding himself in a new place in relation to himself and his patient. Such changes and transformations have been well described in our literature. Here, with this dream and my remembering it in the way that I did, I am fully living in my patient's world as I "dream" that world. And in so dreaming it, I allow myself to feel, in experiential form, the mystery of human drama, conflict, and fear. But most importantly, from the point of view I have been espousing in this chapter, my dreaming and remembering the dreaming both demonstrate and create a new and emerging subjective/emotional/analytic position in relation to my patient Thomas, in relation to his specific human drama and conflict, to his "world" and his "life." In this dream I see my own "dream work," in that I have found myself in a place I didn't know I could inhabit but now did: that place not only of the "politically incorrect," but on that knife's edge of danger and fear in the face of the threat of violence and potential death. Within this dream scene I fully buy into the sense of danger and potential harm that Thomas lives with every waking moment. I also more thoroughly appreciate that I feel a muted form of the danger, captured in the dream, with Thomas in my office, as we are together talking. I am not only afraid *for* him from his first-person position, I am also afraid *of* him from mine. This is of great analytic importance: my more consciously engaging with the domain of fear within the unfolding of our relationship will help me help him be more open to being with that fear as it shows itself in the now-and-the-next of our work. In sum, my analytic position in relation to Thomas is changed, or better *is changing*, as I simultaneously appreciate, *après-coup*, that I had been less charitable, more censorious toward him and more fearful about him than I had let myself know, and, through this dream's proleptic force, that I am ever more Thomas's analyst, and less a distanced and removed private citizen (with proclivities and opinions and the like).

## Concluding Thoughts

In this chapter, I have emphasized the proleptic dimension of the psychoanalytic unconscious at the expense of what is commonly emphasized in the literature—that is, the persistence of past conflict on present experience, both in the patient's life and in the transference-countertransference of the analytic work itself. With Thomas, by way of my dreaming experience, I emerge as a fuller, more engaged analytic subject. Finding myself in another place—the "other scene" of danger and conflict—I can inhabit more fully that fearful place that he brings into the analysis as he and I move into the future of new possibility. I am now more experientially familiar with his fear and my fear, a familiarity that has a chance to help Thomas better live with his fear, learn more about its sources, and perhaps attenuate its hold on him. The past is never simply the past, as if it were an entity with mass and weight inhabiting space. It emerges into the now-and-the-next of the work precisely as it is changing. In this case my fear and censoriousness loosen their grip as I come face to face with their presence.

I wish to emphasize the same point regarding Luna. Without doubt, the other side of Luna's laugh, a laugh brought on by her dream and its liberating features (that she is "shutting the door on shutting the door") was her enduring approach to the world, and her unsatisfactory solution to the problem of devastation when found out as being wrong or faulty. If an analysand's perception of self changes, if new possibilities come into view that the patient now envisions, then she is simultaneously leaving behind a previously held view and, to be more completely descriptive, a previous way of being in the world. For Luna, as with many analysands, this previous way of being was not entirely hidden from her. Rather, it was a way of being she bemoaned, lamented, but also could not help but enact. As analysts we aver our belief in a formal structure—something like "character"—that tends to repeat and has causal consequences for the patient's life. These characteristic ways of being generalize or ramify into ongoing experience, turning what is potentially new into the already familiar and known. Learning and change are anathema, as if the future were already inescapably predicted. Though we can never be certain, it seems entirely plausible that the requisite analytic groundwork had been laid over the six years of treatment from which the "Shut the door, Roberta" dream one day bore fruit, that allowed that dream to be proleptically effective in the way that it was for Luna.

There is a fundamental difference between anticipation and prediction. The proleptic unconscious anticipates, it presents an unfolding vista of new possibility to the subject through a scene both surprising and often contingent—a scene that is received by the subject and transforms him or her, however slightly, then and there, into a way of being hitherto only dimly imagined. Such a picture, and such a transformation, could not have been predicted; neither can it easily be ignored. Prediction, by contrast, arises from the previous, from the past and the history and conflicts that constitute it; it amounts to the expectation of the same. The proleptic unconscious is about the new, the not-yet.

# 10

# "And Let Me Go On": Desire and the Ending of Analysis

*The analyst's desire is directed toward an openness to human passion and suffering that calls for no closure. Yet, all psychoanalyses will, either of necessity or naturally, come to an end. If desire is inexhaustible, then how do we conceptualize the ending of a psychoanalysis? What is the basis of an ethics of psychoanalytic practice in which the analyst's care for the other is primary, along with an ear attuned to the vagaries of desire in both analyst and patient, when it appears that such a practice encourages its ongoingness? This concluding chapter is framed by the metaphor of the inn and its keeper: the patient comes to visit the analyst until he decides to visit her no more.*

*For now had come that moment, that hesitation when dawn trembles and night pauses, when if a feather alight in the scale it will be weighed down. One feather, and the house, sinking, falling, would have turned and pitched downwards to the depths of darkness. In the ruined room, picnickers would have lit their kettles; lovers sought shelter there, lying on the bare boards; and the shepherd stored his dinner on the bricks, and the tramp slept with his coat round him to ward off the cold. Then the roof would have fallen.*
—Virginia Woolf, "Time Passes"

## The Innkeeper, Again

My office flooded a few years ago after the water heater broke. Water wreaks havoc, and in this case, it had found its way nearly everywhere, into the most obscure and precious places where I work and where patients come to visit me, and into the room where they wait prior to these visits. To put things back together such that my office looked like my office again first entailed taking it all apart. Everything of value that could be salvaged needed a safe perch. The analytic couch and various chairs and my desk had to be set on blocks to dry out. Because mold threatens all things wet, carpeting and baseboards (and some books and files) had to be taken up and either entirely discarded or carefully desiccated by a dehumidifying fan that blew day and night for a week. I saw firsthand, right there, that my work-space, that place where I and my patients lay it on the line every day, is constructed, highly fabricated, because it can so easily be deconstructed, even destroyed. "One feather," as Woolf writes, and "the roof would have fallen."

As I wrote in Chapter 2, analysis is based on a handshake, a set of agreements regarding the conditions under which the patient comes to visit the analyst. If there is no place to do this visiting—no physical structure to house those who chose to engage with each other in the project of speaking suffering in order to change its form—then there is no psychoanalysis.

Eventually, for every analyst and every analysand, no matter how sturdy and resilient the structure, there will be no more psychoanalysis. Buildings tend to outlive their occupants, as did the Ramsay House on the Isle of Skye in *To the Lighthouse*. In "Time Passes," the brief middle section of the novel, we're told that Mrs. Ramsay had died suddenly in her sleep, that Andrew Ramsay was killed in the Great War, and that Prue Ramsay had passed from complications of child birth. All this news is brought to us in the unceremonious dress of parentheses.

The empty and unvisited house is the main character in these pages. It lists, and creaks, and moans through the seasons, year after year. Rains batter it; sunlight parches it; winds make it tremble. All of this Woolf renders weirdly, in language that is profuse and lovely, severe and unsparing. We become fascinated with a dwelling that had been so full of life years before, and that now approaches nearly skeletal decay. Clearly, everything that people construct will fall apart, eventually.

But there is, after all, a narrative trick at play that allows us to be in a place where no one actually is: the narrator, in the guise of "certain airs, detache[s] from the body of the wind (the house was ramshackle after all), cre[eps] round corners and venture[s] in doors" ([1927] 1981, 125). So disembodied, we venture, drifting slowly through the house, taking our time, as we become intimate with, as Charles Baxter says, all the "talking forks" (2008, 74–9), the various objects that take on ghostly life. Rusty saucepans and threadbare mats, moving shadows on flapping wallpaper, creaky hinges, old shoes, an errant floorboard come loose, an unruly garden all overgrown— these are what we see as we drift from room to room. At the same time, we are—like the spirit of God in the Hebrew Bible—everywhere at once; we inhabit the house in its entirety, forever grateful for this opportunity to be where no one else is. It does, in fact, feel miraculous that we are here in the old Ramsay abode! ... here where, in the past, many were. In that past, as we know from the book's first section, "The Window," moments of intense feeling and thought took place, while nothing by way of conventional action happened at all.

We have no such narrative luxury in psychoanalysis. We can't be where we are not. We remember and ponder, obviously, those who are not present, those who are not where we happen to be. We may make them present by way of consciously intended recollection, or at times we suffer their company in unbidden dream images and scenes that often take us completely aback. ("I had no *idea* that I had been thinking about him or wondering about her.") All the people I have seen in my office over these past thirty years, where did they go? Where are they now? How are they doing? *What* are they doing? I mean at this very moment. I think of many of them, from time to time. A few I think about on a daily basis. What do they think about? Who among them is gone?

The space in which the analyst works is as precious as it is temporary. At some point in the future, the analyst will no longer work there. Someone else will take it over and do with it what she will. The voice may endure, and the mind braids together the threads of reminiscences, but only as long as the body on which they depend continues going on being.

## "And Let Me Go On"

Once a patient told me about a friend who was also in psychoanalysis. By my patient's telling, his friend had been in analysis for close to a decade and had felt grateful to her analyst for the work they had done. During a recent session her analyst, knowing that he, the analyst, was bringing up a charged and potentially difficult topic, asked his patient: "How long do you imagine or want to continue to meet?" The patient replied (again, as reported to me by my patient): "As long as we can, if not forever."

This story was, in part, told to me by someone who himself had made it clear that ending analysis with me was, at times, unthinkable. And yet, both of us knew that at some point our work together would end, if only because lives, at some point or other, end. He wanted to know—and it took some gentle coaxing on my part for him plainly to ask me—where I thought he and I "were at" in our work together. It was a big moment, as we more directly broached a subject that we had hitherto avoided. I told him that the feeling I had about where we were at in this analysis, in this relationship, was "in the middle" of things. "We're in a vast middle," I said. "That's the sense I have. It's much more a feeling than an assessment or a judgment. Our work has been meaningful and important, for both of us, obviously. We've been through a lot and are the better for it. I know you are freaked out by the thought of ending, or that I want to pull the plug, cut back, or even retire."

How did I arrive at this sense that he and I are "in the middle" of our work together? Often as I am listening to a patient I have spatial images that show up in my mind: a field that is colored, demarcated, empty, or weighed down in some area of it; or a container ship filled with cargo coming into (or perhaps leaving) harbor; or a cookie jar brimming with freshly baked cookies. These are a few of the images that have recently come to mind as I listen. Usually I find a way to describe the image to the patient in the hope that it helps us give shape—to "formulate," to use Donnel Stern's important idea—what the patient is gesturing toward, wondering or worrying about. Sometimes patients take up what I make explicit is *my* offering, and at other times they don't. This giving shape to experience, and finding ways to speak to these images and the experiences they represent, is part of the proleptic engagement—this leaning forward into the future with this image now in tow—that I wrote about in Chapter 9. In the case of my feeling "in the middle," I did not have an image that came to me. Instead, I had a distinctly bodily sensation that was itself distinctly spatial: of sitting in my chair "in the middle"—that is, not listing or leaning to the left or the right. In giving thought to this feeling, I realize now (as I write this) that implicitly or procedurally the "left" is toward the beginning of the analysis, and the "right" would signify its end.[1] The feeling of sitting alertly poised—not troping in any direction—itself felt right. "This is where we are, as best I can tell," I said. "What's your feeling about it?" He replied: "This is the best relationship I've ever had. I don't want it to end."

Many years ago, I published a paper, "'and let me go on'—*Tristram Shandy*, Lacanian Theory, and the Dialectic of Desire" (Wilson 1986). There I offered a close reading of that great comic novel. Also, I argued that the structure of the novel (as well as its thematic preoccupations) and the basic structure of Lacanian theory were isomorphic: fearful of closure and, ultimately, death, both Lacan and Tristram/*Tristram* not only privileged desire, but idealized it. Desire is "indestructible" according to Lacan, following Freud. In my *Tristram* paper I called this claim into question:

---

[1] Perhaps this sense of "left to right," "beginning to end," is connected to reading procedures in English. If I were a native speaker of Hebrew, by contrast, would I sense within the spatial relations of my body that the right is the beginning and the left the end?

It is not only Tristram but more surprisingly, Lacan—Tristram's modern, if somewhat refracted, mirror image—who writes and speaks in the spirit of the "fictive," who contributes to a "literature" the primary move of which is one of the imagination: where Desire runs free and its death is perpetually invoked only to be perpetually deferred. (1986, 370)

Desire, as idealized, is the last lure of the Imaginary.

I want to pull back some from this critique. What I wrote thirty years ago may still be a compelling argument within the domain of literary criticism, but I don't think it tallies with my experience as a psychoanalyst. Lacan was onto something extremely important regarding desire and its various itineraries. Like running water that overflows its vessel and pursues the most expedient downhill path—as I learned from my broken water heater—desire will find its way through the cracks and crevices of any structure or bulwark. Desire's "containment" is always partial; it will forever "go on." Corporal Trim's flourish with his stick comes yet again to mind in this regard (see Fig. 1, Chapter 2).

In the rest of this chapter I want to consider the question of desire and its "indestructability" especially as it relates to whether it is possible *to stop doing* analytic work. My patient, and his friend, both wish to be in analysis "forever." I feel that he and I are "in a vast middle," something like the middle of an unending ocean. To get to land, in whatever direction, could take an eternity. In *Tristram Shandy*, Tristram, forever afraid of castration and death, bids the God Priapus to "let me go on." Lacan says that Freud says that desire never dies. And not only do some analysands want the analysis to go on forever, some analysts do too. They like being analysts, and at times they love being analysts with certain patients. Further, the analyst's gyroscopic position, and the futural, anticipatory nature of the proleptic unconscious, also suggest that the psychoanalytic project, the very human machinery that makes it go, simply is built to keep going. If, as Stern (2018) has intimated, there exists the "infinity of the unsaid," in which what is at stake is the yet-to-be-formulated, the yet-to-be-realized, then there is always more to give shape to and actualize in psychoanalysis. One cannot subtract something from infinity and thereby lessen its reach.

With these thoughts now present before us, what is an ethics of psychoanalysis that takes seriously this question of the "forever" nature of analytic desire? How do we think about the question of endings—their very possibility—in relation to this question of "forever"? The issue is difficult to think through and offers no straightforward answer, as it can easily lead to pronouncements and claims that end in narcissistic cul-de-sacs and idealizations.[2] There is also embedded in this question an irresolvable conflict between the logic of desire (as I said, the "human machinery" that makes it all go), and conventional professional practice of most any kind in which a discrete presenting problem is addressed by a specific and targeted service intended to solve it. Once solved, the service is no longer needed.[3]

## The Psychoanalyst as Fetishized Object

Though, or perhaps because, this conflict is truly irresolvable, the interminability of some analyses has worried analysts even before Freud wrote his last great paper, "Analysis Terminable and Interminable" (1937). Years earlier Ferenczi said: "The proper ending of an analysis is when neither the physician nor the patient puts an end to it, but when it dies of exhaustion, so to speak" ([1927] 1999, 254). More recently, Owen Renik (1992) and Irwin Hirsch (2008) have explicitly and pointedly addressed treatments that seem to go on forever. They especially highlight the shaky ethical substrate upon which such analytic work rests. Perhaps it's easier for the analyst just to "coast" (to use Hirsch's damning phrase) than to do the difficult work of ending. This work of ending may involve, as Renik emphasizes, confronting the patient about his willful blurring of fantasy and reality, a blurring that Renik links to faulty superego functioning in the patient. Regarding the analyst, she may be reluctant to do such work, and is instead perversely gratified by being "fetishized" by the patient. The analytic relationship, in this case, is based on an unexamined "illusion" (Renik's word)—that is, an insistence that the analyst has something the patient doesn't have and will never obtain. Lacan, as I mentioned in the Preface, came to conceptualize the entirety of the transference as caused by this fantasy: the analyst has a special something, shiny and precious, that the patient wishes to extract from her. He called this, variously, *das Ding*, the *agalma*, and finally *objet petit a*.[4] The analyst is not seen as a desiring being that is necessarily lacking (symbolically castrated), but instead is imagined to possess a magical substance that obscures the

---

[2] I have in mind descriptions of "terminations" that emphasize the patient's identification with the analyst, and that, further, stress the role of mourning and the integration of the personality. I will not discuss these issues in this chapter.

[3] In this chapter I am not discussing the various practical issues—most notably time and money—that almost always are at play regarding the ending of any given psychotherapy or analysis.

[4] In his seminar *Anxiety*, Lacan ([1962–3] 2014) describes the intensity of the patient's attempt at what he termed the "sadistic" extraction of this object; see especially his discussion of Lucia Tower's classic paper, "Countertransference" (1956), 191–7.

reality of this condition. This illusory relationship conspires against the analyst addressing with the patient this very illusion. Renik writes:

> When an analyst, wittingly or unwittingly, allows himself or herself to be used as a fetish, the treatment becomes interminable. The patient remains forever dependent, a "lifer" of one kind or another. These clinical situations can always be explained on the basis of the severity of the patient's psychopathology and his or her limited capacity for analytic work, but there is the question of how adequately fetishism within the treatment relationship has been addressed. (557)

The view of proper analytic work alluded to here—that is, to find ways to address fetishism within and of the treatment relationship—entails the pursuit of so-called objective truth, the gradual improvement of the patient's reality testing (distinguishing fantasy from reality), and the letting go of "illusions," because the patient comes to acknowledge these are false and are inhibiting the living of a fuller life. This rather classical view emerges from a clear trend in Freud: that the patient comes to us suffering from the living out of a confusion or mistake, that of mixing up internal, wishful exigencies with external facts and states of affairs. If this is how the patient's fundamental problem is conceived, then psychoanalytic work is in an important sense cognitive: the patient gains insight into these confusions; crooked thinking is straightened out, including the patient's mixing up the illusory nature of the analytic relationship with a "real" one. But in so-called interminable cases in which the patient fetishizes the analyst, such work is averred by the analyst not to be possible. This is because of the "severity of the patient's psychopathology."

Renik sets up particularly well the terms and territory of this question of desire and interminability: are all analyses that go on and on necessarily false, ethically questionable, and ultimately damaging to the patient's autonomy and capacities for change? In such a circumstance, is the patient *always* caught within the lure of a fetishized object, the *agalma*, the *objet a*? An object that, in point of fact, exists only as a stopgap against absence? Clearly, this is possible and is a psychoanalytic dead end. The analyst must not only be on the alert for such a state of affairs but also be willing to address it with the patient. But this would be a very tall order to pull off if the analyst is seen as a heroic figure—indispensable—and perhaps a messianic one. This view can come from the patient, analyst, or be mutually shared. It may be explicitly understood between the parties, or unconsciously believed or wished for by either one or both. Some writing in our literature tends to encourage this view that something magical is happening and is mutually shared, as the analyst tends to be described as a two-dimensional maternal figure, ever-present and available, empathic (if not endlessly so), fulfilling necessary functions (holding, containing, and the like) that the patient lacks. The patient, as lacking, tends to be seen as burdened by severe psychopathology that supports as a kind of clinical justification the analyst's position as savior. The patient is said to have faulty symbolic capacities and to be haunted by split-off parts of the self, or grappling with "unrepresented mental states." Regarding any given patient this all may, in some sense, be the case; but as I described in Chapter 9, there is the ever-present tendency to reify, as Freud said, "the figurative language peculiar to psychology." To the extent that the analyst's role is conceptualized as primarily supplying capacities that the patient lacks, this set-up risks the analyst's inhabiting a position as the "healthy" one and the giver of necessary "provisions." These are examples of narcissistic cul-de-sacs that I mentioned earlier. They are contemporary versions of the analyst as the one who "knows."

## Illusion and the Real

Analytic thought about these issues has evolved substantially since Renik wrote his challenge to what he saw as a disturbing trend in psychoanalytic practice.[5] I will, near the end of this chapter, return to this vexing question of the analyst as an object of fetishistic fascination and its role, or not, in ongoing analyses. Here I want to take up a related question that has both interpersonal and more unconscious aspects. Is the analytic relationship illusory? Is it not real life? It seems to me that we have clear answers to these questions and they are noncontroversial: the analytic relationship is not illusory. The analytic relationship is real life. Further, illusion is an important ingredient in any analysis. Illusion, in other words, is real and is not to be viewed entirely with suspicion, because illusion is not something we can do without (nor, in my view, would we wish to do without it). In short, the fantasy-reality distinction Renik relies on becomes, in contemporary writing, much more complex.

Two analysts who are especially helpful on this question of illusion are Stephen Seligman and Humphrey Morris. Seligman, building on Winnicott's

---

[5] It is notable how little information we have about how analysts actually practice, including whether analyses are longer, generally speaking, or shorter, or whatever. All I can say here is that in my experience analyses seem to me to be longer. Even when external circumstances intervene, like a relocation because of a job change, the therapeutic work tends to be carried on over the internet or the phone.

central notion of transitional phenomena, calls the human capacity for illusion the "third principle of mental functioning" (along with the pleasure and reality principles). Our capacity for illusion is what allows us to light the myriad objects we find in the world with sense and color. Seligman (2018) writes:

> Illusion … is as fundamental a psychological dynamic and form as fantasy, defense, projection, adaptation, attachment, and others prominent in the analytic canon, but distinct from them. Illusion carries the energy, as it were, of the mind's reach into the world, investing it with meaning and affective salience—feeling and engagement in their broader senses. (265)

Seligman captures well that illusion exists in a dialectical relation to disillusion, and while he grants as obvious that human development involves a gradual movement from illusion (e.g., omnipotent fantasy) to disillusion (i.e., reality-based cognition), he shows that in the most "adult" of activities— whether it be attending a play, falling in love, avidly following a sports team, or being a patient in psychoanalysis—illusion brings these endeavors to life, vivifies them, lights them up.

Morris, while leaning heavily on Laplanche and only secondarily on Winnicott, has a remarkably similar take on the issue of illusion as the one Seligman offers us. But Morris is more pointed and incisive, perhaps reflective of the hard-nosed rigor of Laplanche's approach to psychoanalytic theory and practice. Not only does Morris agree that psychoanalytic experience— the relationship, the engagement and commitment, the wishful loose talk— is ontologically real, but he also has a clear-eyed view of just how real the analytic situation is: "Psychoanalysis is a practice of living the real at the level of our basic existential situation in relation to one another. The ethics of psychoanalysis, most primally, is the ethics of a human encounter that stages both new possibilities of intimacy and new necessities of separateness" (2016, 1174–5).

Imagine the following clinical moment, one that in its countless manifestations is well-known to almost any analyst: a patient brings the analyst a gift and the analyst accepts it. In this particular analysis, this gift-giving is occasional and the analyst always receives it graciously. Following these exchanges, the analyst thanks the patient and asks about the patient's experience of the exchange and the backstory of giving this gift on this day. Often the entire interchange is simply part of the ongoingness of the work, but on this day the analyst does something with the card that accompanied the gift that immediately upsets the patient, who acutely and perceptively notices a hesitation on the analyst's part. To the patient, this hesitation—so slight as to be nearly invisible—is temporarily upending: "You're trying to hide something from me, but I can see what you did." And this feeling of great disturbance is only temporary because the analyst recognizes and acknowledges that she did something upsetting to the patient that can't be taken away, whether by rational explanation or by some other equally false means.

Analysts have learned not to pretend such moments away by ignoring them or rationalizing them with various interpretive maneuvers, the most well-worn of which is the "transference interpretation"—that the patient, in other words, is "enacting" or "repeating" an internal conflict or fantasy in the room with the analyst. Instead, the analyst finds ways to speak to these moments, or rather, to speak to the patient about such moments. For the analyst, this is an entirely singular speaking, in her own voice, that the patient comes to know and to trust (though, as I have just described, this trust has its limits). It is rather more complex than this, because the analyst is as much speaking to herself and to the analytic couple qua dyad, as she is to the patient as other person. In some ways we might say that in moments such as this the analyst is "tending the field," amending the analytic soil with the analyst's desire, with human essentials such as kindness, patience, and a speaking that strives to capture something of the truth of what is transpiring, all of which encompasses how the analytic relationship *is* living the real.

But this aspect of psychoanalytic work, that is, *the real, the actual*—one whose importance cannot be emphasized enough—includes the embrace of illusion as part of its core. Illusion-as-reality is not to be interpreted or otherwise explained away. Innumerable are the means by which analytic experience can be dismissed as false and unreal, including the question of the analyst's dedication, caring, and love for the analysand. Here we again confront the question of the complexity of the analyst's ethical position, her desire as analyst, which trenches on the nature of the analyst's love, what Lawrence Friedman calls the "flickering apparition of the analyst's deep and lasting attachment to the patient" (quoted in Morris 2016, 1175). This flickering apparition is evocative of the fetishistic object, its veiled presence, and the question of its ontological existence: does the analyst love me unconditionally, unequivocally? Is this love indelible? Is it in the real or in my mind? As Friedman emphasizes, the analyst's love flickers; it is both there and not there. Morris points out, in a way that cannot be gainsaid, that this very apparition, this "deep and lasting attachment," is central to living the real of psychoanalysis:

> As if the thing we call real life were not based on just such illusions [i.e., the "flickering apparition ..."]. No, let's be honest: unconscious process

and fantasy notwithstanding, analysis is not as-if life, not a pretend or metaphorical or virtual version of some other life that can reliably be taken as a stable extrinsic point of reference, be that other life life in the outside world or the life of unconscious drives. (1175)

We have here a paradox that is not only semantic: the analyst's love is both real and an illusion, and a constitutive part of its reality is its illusory quality. At the center of this paradox sits Laplanche's "enigma," the enigma of the analyst's desire, which the analyst struggles as best she can to be with so its liveliness, its vivifying energy, does not get closed down or snuffed out (reduced, that is, to a version of "reality").

But from another point of view, things are better defined; they are not at all enigmatic. There is, as I've described in several places along the way, an essential asymmetry in the analytic relationship, in that the analyst's desire is orthogonal to the patient's wishes. This asymmetry is captured in the fact that the analyst does not, as a general matter, give patients gifts. Nor does the analyst pay the patient for his or her services. These facts are among the many constitutive disavowals of the analytic relationship, structural features of psychoanalysis that are very real.

We can now circle back to the question of desire and the seeming interminability of psychoanalysis. As I said earlier in this chapter, there are many facets to this question. For starters, what if—contra the fetishized analyst in therapies that appear stuck—the analysand describes improvement in his or her outside life, and, further, the analytic relationship deepens over time? Though the analysis might, here and there, appear stuck, a larger view (the "ends of analysis" view I wrote about in Chapter 8) allows the analyst to see that transformation, however slow, is occurring. Both patient and analyst evolve and change, and the analyst evolves for the benefit of the patient. Recall Kravis's description: "It might be fair to say that some analyses take a very long time because it takes the analyst a long time to become that patient's analyst" (2017, 800). Both parties are better able to be with each other in the room during sessions, including an increased ability to tolerate and talk about the ways in which the analyst has been helpful or disappointing or hurtful to the patient.[6] In short, not uncommonly one sees demonstrable progress in a patient who wishes to be in analysis "forever." The patient wants to continue in analysis for any number of reasons, one of which is that it is importantly, perhaps singularly, helpful.

---

[6] Talking about how the analyst has been helpful can be just as, or more, difficult than discussing hurtful moments as I describe at the end of Chapter 8.

More difficult to think through are issues captured in my patient's statement that his relationship with me was the "best" he had ever had. And here, certainly, we can understand the caution that Renik and Hirsch both give voice to, that the analytic relationship, for all its "realness," remains a contrived or constructed relationship, one that develops within a specific professional frame that includes the exchange of payment for services rendered, all for the purpose of the patient's well-being and growth. The claim in this case would be that the analytic relationship, when seen for what it "truly" is (contrived, professional, and the like), *cannot be* on par with intimate relationships outside of the consulting room. But again, it seems to me, we find ourselves in the same fantasy-reality binary that we were a few pages ago, only now burdened with a further confusion, a misreading of the basic nature of all human interacting and relating: all of it is contrived in some way. Not only is the analyst's office constructed, literally, of wood and nails and plaster, but its status as a legitimate space in which to conduct professional work is also dependent upon a variety of legal agreements, property ownership, and a state-sponsored clinical license. All social engagements of any kind are based on accepted conventions and background assumptions that give meaning to what transpires, from having an intimate conversation with one's partner or close friend to buying food at the local market. It's not as if what I am writing here, the purposes I have for it, the audience I am intending to reach, as well as the words and the ways I am putting them together on this page—that all of it is not bound by and made meaningful because of a complex set of conventions and agreements. This is always the case. It is simply that the analytic relationship has its own set of conventions and agreements, its own rules of the game, its own constitutive disavowals and acknowledgments.

We now come to the heart of the matter, something that we know makes some analysts quite uneasy: the psychoanalytic relationship *is* like no other in a patient's life. And the psychoanalytic relationship is like no other in the analyst's life. Freud gestures in this direction when he writes: "The course the analyst must pursue is ... one for which there is no model in real life" (1915, 166). Freud is discussing how the analyst ought to proceed with a patient who appears to be in love with him. My emphasis is on the analytic relationship more generally, and for that there *is* no model in real life.

We have, then, an eminently real relationship that is sui generis, literally incomparable, entirely its own animal, with protections and structuring that allow for an especially intimate intimacy. So when my patient says, "This is the best relationship I have ever had," we must take him at his word. There is a very real sense in which this is a true statement. In no other ongoing human engagement that I know of is it ethically incumbent upon the people involved to speak truthfully to each other, with this further feature: the relationship is fundamentally asymmetrical in several important ways, one of which is that the analyst attends as responsibly as she can to the nuances of the interaction and especially to its disruptions. Of course, at times the analyst fails in this task of attentiveness, as the analyst can never be entirely, one-hundred percent attentive. This is clearly true. Nor would we want it *not* to be true. The choreography and rhythms of human engagement would be thoroughly disrupted by the analyst's being ever-present. This iterative, recursive effort—this fading and coming back—is itself of great importance to the patient and has, all its own, significant therapeutic value.

For an increasing number of analysts, clinical work is viewed as *indistinguishable* from the qualities of the relationship that develops as the patient comes to visit the analyst over a number of years. We would even say, ca. 2020, that the analytic relationship as it unfolds, as it moves proleptically into the future, *is* the work. Obviously, the qualities of this relationship—its aliveness, vibrancy, and resilience in the face of the bumps and bruises, the dead spaces and desultory periods, that will invariably occur—are necessary conditions for something truly therapeutic to happen. What I am saying here follows directly from my discussion in Chapter 2 (the analyst is an innkeeper) of the grounding conditions of the *matricial* for all that transpires in a psychoanalysis, and also the analyst's *gyroscopic* position that I described in relation to the analyst's lack and ongoing desire in Chapter 5. The speech relation, as I have emphasized, instantiates this proleptic movement, in that the degrees of freedom within the speech act allow for something new to emerge in the now-and-the-next of the work.

Where do insight and understanding fit within this contemporary view? Insight as the salve for errant thinking based on fantasy, illusion, and the like has a decidedly uncertain status. In fact, I think that it is quite the wrong word, if by insight we mean "seeing into" or "apprehending the nature of things." Here we lurch back to the view of "the" unconscious housing concretized contents: split off selves and various forms of conflict and fantasy. Even with aspects of the proleptic unconscious, in which a shift in attention immediately transforms the subject, the analyst, or the field into an altered futural space or position, so-called prior mental content (conflicts, dispositions) is neither disclosed nor revealed so much as *something new is being made*, is given expressible form. Insight in the conventional psychoanalytic sense may be a byproduct of this work in that felt truths can take shape, but it is not the main event in most psychoanalyses I have been a part of or have heard colleagues discuss in study groups and the like. As I have argued throughout this book, the analyst is not the giver of knowledge; she is the facilitator of the unrealized coming into being, and so she is the curator, even the midwife of space. To quote Robert Hunter again: "His job is to shed light, not to master." He (or she), obviously, is the analyst.

## The Enduring Logic of Psychoanalytic Work

Yes, the analytic relationship is real. Yes, the analytic relationship involves, constitutively and structurally, disavowals and acknowledgments. Yes, the analyst's desire must be meaningfully engaged to motivate the entire enterprise, especially its ethical core, in dialectical fashion, iteratively, over time. And yes, taken together, the analytic relationship is sui generis, entirely its own thing, and is, for some, the best relationship they have ever had.

And yet, the best relationship is by no means a perfect one. There is nothing to idealize about this "best." An inherent feature of this best is that psychoanalysis can at times feel horrible. The especially intimate intimacy that psychoanalysis aims to engender makes what can happen if things "going south in a hurry" (as I described in Chapter 2) exquisitely painful. The analyst is well-versed in the horrible, well-versed in this particular kind of pain, having had her own experience of these feelings in her analysis. As we know, her ethical responsibility is to stay fully in the room with the patient during these moments, gyroscopically to "roll" with them. This is the key element in an ethically based psychoanalytic praxis: that the analyst is "at-one" with these moments, and "knows" that they are a vital, if disturbing, part of what makes psychoanalysis potentially transformative for the patient (and, of necessity, for the analyst). In fact, a key element of this "best" is that the analyst is, in her open, futural, gyroscopic orientation, always, sometimes explicitly but always implicitly (i.e., to herself) taking responsibility for her impactful desire as best she can, an effort that is always partial.

This is the essential logic of the analytic project: it is built to keep going because the analyst's desire is directed toward an openness to human passion and suffering that calls for no closure. The idea that illusions are seen to be what they truly are, and the enduring "patterns" and conflicts are eventually given up, is a remnant of a psychopathological therapeutics that runs the great risk of reinforcing that which one wants to get rid of. The patient's relationship to his suffering may change; the suffering itself rarely does. The giving up of a symptom, as Gabbard and Ogden (2010) have wisely cautioned, ought not be unthinkingly adopted as a primary goal of an analysis. Lacan came to the same conclusion with his theory of the *sinthome*. But this question of the role of the symptom in psychoanalysis must be left for another time.

## The Visitor Leaves the Innkeeper

When Ferenczi writes that "the proper ending of an analysis is when neither the physician nor the patient puts an end to it, but when it dies of exhaustion, so to speak" ([1927] 1999, 254), he is capturing something about the nature of desire in psychoanalysis that feels true. But the ways in which this dying of exhaustion comes about cannot be scripted or choreographed in advance. It's infinitely easier if, as is usually the case, practical concerns intervene, which can turn the question of ending into a utilitarian calculus: is the analysis worth the money, or time, or distance to continue? Ferenczi's "proper ending" suggests that something quite apart from the practical does change, something internal to the patient in relation to the analyst. The analyst's giving of her desire—to listen, to care, and inhabit a lacking, gyroscopic position—doesn't cease. The door to her office is, metaphorically speaking, always open. And yet, the patient's position in relation to the analyst's desire changes in some meaningful sense. Here perhaps Lacan is right, after all. Perhaps the patient has both gotten things good and valuable from the analyst and the analysis, and also has come to feel that enough is enough, that the veil in some sense has fallen from his eyes, that—to evoke the Maltese falcon again—there is nothing there beyond the analyst's basic humanity.

But the patient would have great difficulty leaving if the analyst is seen or experienced as a full presence, heroic, messianic—as really possessing that special something the patient feels he lacks. In such a case, either the patient believes he can't live without the analyst, or he imagines that the analyst, behind the image of full presence, is actually quite weak and vulnerable and so the patient feels unconsciously protective of her. Certainly, the analyst has a clear responsibility to address this state of affairs. But the fact is that to do so successfully does not mean that the patient would wish, as a consequence of this talk, to end the analysis. Quite the contrary may be true.

Psychoanalysis begins with the analyst's offer of analysis: "I would like to see you several days a week." The visitor says yes, and so becomes a patient. The analysis ends when the patient decides to visit the analyst no more. They say goodbye to each other one last time, perhaps with a handshake, or with a hug, or with a simple nod of the head. "Good luck," the analyst says. "Let me know how things go, if you want to." "I will. And thank you." The patient leaves. The sound of his footsteps fades as he walks away and into the distance. And maybe that's it. Maybe that's all she wrote. Maybe not. But at that moment the analyst is left to ponder what just transpired—the years of hard work, of talking and grappling with the difficult and the impossible.

Unlike the ubiquity of the narrator in a work of fiction in which even empty houses can be inhabited—in which, that is, we can be where we are not—in psychoanalysis, the analyst cannot be where she is not. The patient has gone to live his life and she is alone. What does the analyst do now? The afternoon sun angles through the window as she tidies up, and then sits in silence for some minutes, or makes a phone call or two. Perhaps she readies herself for her next visitor.

# References

Aguayo, J. (2017), Review of *The Complete Works of W. R. Bion*, *International Journal of Psychoanalysis*, 98: 221–43.

Akerlof, G. (1970), "A Market for Lemons," *Quarterly Journal of Economics*, 84: 488–500.

Almond, R. (1995), "The Analytic Role," *Journal of the American Psychoanalytic Association*, 43: 469–94.

Altieri, C. (1996), "The Values of Articulation: Aesthetics after the Aesthetic Ideology," in *Beyond Representation: Philosophy and Poetic Imagination*, ed. Richard Eldridge, Cambridge: Cambridge University Press, 66–89.

Altieri, C. (2015), *Reckoning with the Imagination: Wittgenstein and the Aesthetics of Literary Experience*, Ithaca, NY: Cornell University Press.

Annas, J. (1993), *The Morality of Happiness*, New York: Oxford University Press.

Arlow, J. A. (1969), "Unconscious Fantasy and Disturbances in Conscious Experience," *Psychoanalytic Quarterly*, 38: 1–27.

Arlow, J. A. (1995), "Stilted Listening: Psychoanalysis as Discourse," *Psychoanalytic Quarterly*, 64: 215–33.

Aron, L. (2006), "Analytic Impasse and the Third: Clinical Implications of Intersubjectivity Theory," *International Journal of Psychoanalysis*, 87: 349–68.

Austin, J. L. (1962), *How to Do Things with Words*, Cambridge, MA: Harvard University Press.

Balliett, W. (1976), "Big Sid," *New Yorker*, March 8.

Baranger, M., Baranger, W., and Mom, J. (1983), "Process and Non-process in Analytic Work," *International Journal of Psychoanalysis*, 64: 1–15.

Barthes, R. (1977), *Image-Music-Text*, London: Fontana.

Baxter, C. (2008), *Burning Down the House, Expanded Edition*, Saint Paul, MN: Gray Wolf.

Beebe, B. (2014), "My Journey in Infant Research and Psychoanalysis: Microanalysis, a Social Microscope," *Psychoanalytic Psychology*, 31: 4–25.

Benjamin, J. (1988), *The Bonds of Love: Psychoanalysis, Feminism, and the Problem of Domination*, New York: Pantheon.

Benjamin, J. (2000), "The Shadow of the Other Subject: Intersubjectivity and Feminist Theory," in *Psychoanalysis at Its Limits: Navigating the Post-Modern Turn*, ed. C. Spezzano and A. Elliott, London: Free Association Books, 79–109.

Benjamin, J. (2004), "Beyond Doer and Done to: An Intersubjective View of Thirdness," *Psychoanalytic Quarterly*, 73: 5–46.

Benvenuto, B. and Kennedy, R. (1986), *The Works of Jacques Lacan: An Introduction*, New York: St. Martin's.

Bion, W. R. (1959), "Attacks on Linking," *International Journal of Psychoanalysis*, 40: 308–15.

Bion, W. R. (1970), *Attention and Interpretation*, London: Karnac.
Bion, W. R. (1988), "Notes on Memory and Desire," in *Melanie Klein Today: Developments in Theory and Practice. Volume 2: Mainly Practice*, ed. E. B. Spillius, London: Routledge, 17–21.
Bion, W. R. (1994), *Clinical Seminars and Other Works*, London: Karnac.
Bion, W. R. (2005), *The Italian Seminars*, trans. P. Slotkin, London: Routledge.
Bion, W. R. (2013), *Los Angeles Seminars and Supervision*, ed. J. Aguayo and B. Malin, London: Karnac.
Bloom, H. (1975), *Kabbalah and Criticism*, New York: Continuum.
Boesky, D. (1990), "The Psychoanalytic Process and Its Components," *Psychoanalytic Quarterly*, 64: 282–305.
Bollas, C. (1989), *Forces of Destiny: Psychoanalysis and Human Idiom*, London: Free Association Books.
Brenman-Pick, I. (1985), "Working-through in the Countertransference," *International Journal of Psychoanalysis*, 66: 157–66.
Britton, R. and Steiner, J. (1994), "Interpretation: Selected Fact or Overvalued Idea?" *International Journal of Psychoanalysis*, 75: 1069–78.
Browning, R. ([1842] 1993), *My Last Duchess and Other Poems*, Mineola, NY: Dover.
Busch, F. and Joseph, B. (2004), "A Missing Link in Psychoanalytic Technique: Psychoanalytic Consciousness," *International Journal of Psychoanalysis*, 85: 567–78.
Butler, J. (2005), *Giving an Account of Oneself*, New York: Fordham University Press.
Caper, R. (1997), "A Mind of One's Own," *International Journal of Psychoanalysis*, 78: 265–78.
Carson, A. (1998), *Eros the Bittersweet*, Champaign, IL: Dalkey Archive.
Casement, J. (1985), *Learning from the Patient*, New York: Guilford Press.
Casement, J. (2002), *Learning from Our Mistakes: Beyond Dogma in Psychoanalysis and Psychotherapy*, New York: Guilford Press.
Chappell, S. G. (2015), "Bernard Williams," in *The Stanford Encyclopedia of Philosophy*, ed. E. N. Zalta, retrieved from https://plato.stanford.edu/entries/williams-bernard/ (January 1, 2016).
Chetrit-Vatine, V. (2014), *The Ethical Seduction of the Analytic Situation: The Feminine-Maternal Origins of Responsibility for the Other*, London: Karnac.
Chused, J. F. (1991), "The Evocative Power of Enactments," *Journal of the American Psychoanalytic Association*, 39: 615–40.
Civitarese, G. (2005), "Fire in the Theater: (Un)reality of/in the Transference and Interpretation," *International Journal of Psychoanalysis*, 86: 1299–316.
Civitarese, G. (2016), *Truth and the Unconscious in Psychoanalysis*, Oxford: Routledge.
Cooper, S. (2004), "State of the Hope: The New Bad Object in the Therapeutic Action of Psychoanalysis," *Psychoanalytic Dialogues*, 14: 527–51.

Cooper, S. (2010), *A Disturbance in the Field: Essays in Transference-Countertransference Engagement*, New York: Routledge.
Dunn, J. (1995), "Intersubjectivity in Psychoanalysis: A Critical Review," *International Journal of Psychoanalysis*, 76: 723–38.
Eagle, M. (2010), *From Classical to Contemporary Psychoanalysis: A Critique and Integration*, New York: Routledge.
Eigen, M. ([1981] 1999), "The Area of Faith in Winnicott, Lacan, and Bion," in *Relational Psychoanalysis, Vol. 1: The Emergence of a Tradition*, ed. S. Mitchell and L. Aron, New York: Taylor & Francis, 1–38.
Elise, D. (2019), *Creativity and the Erotic Dimensions of the Analytic Field*, London: Routledge.
Evans, D. (1996), *An Introductory Dictionary of Lacanian Psychoanalysis*, London: Routledge.
Faimberg, H. (1992), "The Countertransference Position and the Countertransference," *International Journal of Psychoanalysis*, 73: 541–7.
Faimberg, H. (1996), "Listening to Listening," *International Journal of Psychoanalysis*, 77: 667–77.
Faimberg, H. (1997), "Misunderstanding and Psychic Truths," *International Journal of Psychoanalysis*, 78: 439–51.
Faimberg, H. (2005), *The Telescoping of Generations: Listening to the Narcissistic Links between Generations*, London: Routledge.
Feldman, M. (1997), "Projective Identification: The Analyst's Involvement," *International Journal of Psychoanalysis*, 78: 227–41.
Feldman, M. (2007), "Racker's Contribution to the Understanding of Countertransference, Revisited," *Psychoanalytic Quarterly*, 76: 779–93.
Ferenczi, S. ([1927] 1999), *Selected Writings*, London: Penguin.
Ferro, A. (2002), *In the Analyst's Consulting Room*, trans. P. Slotkin, East Sussex: Brunner-Routledge.
Fink, B. (1995), *The Lacanian Subject: Between Language and Jouissance*, Princeton, NJ: Princeton University Press.
Fish, S. (1980), *Is There a Text in This Class? The Authority of Interpretive Communities*, Cambridge, MA: Harvard University Press.
Fonagy, P. and Target, M. (1998), "Mentalization and the Changing Aims of Child Psychoanalysis," *Psychoanalytic Dialogues*, 8: 79–87.
Foucault, M. (1977), *Language, Counter-Memory, Practice*, Ithaca, NY: Cornell University Press.
Freud, S. (1900), *The Interpretation of Dreams, The Standard Edition of the Complete Psychological Works of Sigmund Freud*, trans. J. Strachey, London: Hogarth Press and the Institute of Psychoanalysis., 4: 1–338. (Referred to in subsequent references as *S.E.*)
Freud, S. (1914), "On Narcissism," in *S.E.*, trans. J. Strachey, 7: 67–102.
Freud, S. (1915), "Observations on Transference-Love (Further Recommendations on the Technique of Psycho-Analysis)," in *S.E.*, trans.

J. Strachey, London: Hogarth Press and the Institute of Psychoanalysis 12: 157–71.

Freud, S. (1916-17), *Introductory Lectures on Psychoanalysis (Part III)*, S.E., trans. J. Strachey, London: Hogarth Press and the Institute of Psychoanalysis 16: 243–83.

Freud, S. (1920), *Beyond the Pleasure Principle*, S.E., trans. J. Strachey, London: Hogarth Press and the Institute of Psychoanalysis, 18: 1–64.

Freud, S. (1923), *The Ego and the Id*, S.E., trans. J. Strachey, London: Hogarth Press and the Institute of Psychoanalysis, 19: 1–66.

Freud, S. (1927), "Letter to Oskar Pfister," *International Psychoanalytic Library* 59: 117–18.

Freud, S. (1937), "Analysis Terminable and Interminable," in *S.E.*, trans. J. Strachey, London: Hogarth, 23: 209–54.

Freud, S. ([1953] 1986), *The Standard Edition of the Complete Psychological Works of Sigmund Freud*, ed. and trans. J. Strachey et al., 24 vols., London: Hogarth.

Freud, S. (1933), "Dreams and Occultism," in *New Introductory Lectures on Psycho-Analysis, S.E.*, trans. J. Strachey, London: Hogarth Press and the Institute of Psychoanalysis, 22: 31–56.

Freud, S., and Breuer, J. (1895), *Studies in Hysteria*, S.E., trans. J. Strachey, London: Hogarth Press and the Institute of Psychoanalysis, 2.

Friedman, L. (1993), "Discussion, Panel on Resistance in Clinical Practice," American Psychoanalytic Association Annual Meeting, San Francisco, May.

Friedman, L. (2007), "The Delicate Balance of Work and Illusion in Psychoanalysis," *Psychoanalytic Quarterly*, 76: 817–33.

Friedman, L. (2012), "A Holist's Anxiety of Influence: Commentary on Kirshner," *Journal of the American Psychoanalytic Association*, 60: 1259–79.

Fukuyama, F. (1992), "In the Beginning, a Battle to the Death for Pure Prestige," in *The End of History and the Last Man*, New York: Free Press, 143–52.

Gabbard, G. O. (2000), "On Gratitude and Gratification," *Journal of the American Psychoanalytic Association*, 48: 697–716.

Gerson, S. (2004), "The Relational Unconscious: A Core Element of Intersubjectivity, Thirdness, and Clinical Process," *Psychoanalytic Quarterly*, 73: 63–98.

Glover, E. (1931), "The Therapeutic Effect of Inexact Interpretation: A Contribution to the Theory of Suggestion," *International Journal of Psychoanalysis*, 12: 397–411.

Goldberg, A. (2004), *Misunderstanding Freud*, New York: Other Press.

Goldberg, A. (2007), *Moral Stealth: How "Correct Behavior" Insinuates Itself into Clinical Practice*, Chicago, IL: University of Chicago Press.

Goldberg, P. (2012), "Active Perception and the Search for Sensory Symbiosis," *Journal of the American Psychoanalytic Association*, 60: 791–812.

Graves, R. (1955), *The Greek Myths*, vol. 2, Baltimore, MD: Penguin.

Gray, P. (1994), *The Ego and the Analysis of Defense*, New York: Aronson.

Green, A. (1973), "On Negative Capability: A Critical Review of W. R. Bion's Attention and Interpretation," *International Journal of Psychoanalysis*, 54: 115–19.

Green, A. (1975), "The Analyst, Symbolization and Absence in the Analytic Setting (On Changes in Analytic Practice and Analytic Experience)–in Memory of D. W. Winnicott," *International Journal of Psychoanalysis*, 56: 1–22.

Green, A. (1986), *On Private Madness*, Madison, CT: International Universities Press.

Green, A. (1993), *The Work of the Negative*, trans. A. Weller, London: Free Association Books.

Greenberg, J. (1995), "Psychoanalytic Technique and the Interactive Matrix," *Psychoanalytic Quarterly*, 64: 1–22.

Greenberg, J. (2015), "Therapeutic Action and the Analyst's Responsibility," *Journal of the American Psychoanalytic Association*, 63: 15–32.

Greenson, R. R. (2000), "Beginnings: The Preliminary Contacts with the Patient," in *The Technique and Practice of Psychoanalysis, vol. 2: A Memorial Volume to Ralph R. Greenson*, ed. A. Sugarman, R. A. Memiroff, and D. Greenson, New York: International Universities Press, 1–42.

Grossman, L. (1999), "What the Analyst Does Not Hear," *Psychoanalytic Quarterly*, 68: 681–92.

Grossman, W. I. and Simon, B. (1969), "Anthropomorphism–Motive, Meaning, and Causality in Psychoanalytic Theory" in *Psychoanalytic Study of the Child 24*, ed. R. S. Eissler et al., London: Hogarth, 78–111.

Grotstein, J. (1997), "Bion's "Transformation in 'O'" and the Concept of the 'Transcendent Position,'" retrieved from www.sicait/merciai/bion/papers/grots.htm (August 1, 2017).

Harms, D. (2018), "A Shocking Revelation," in *Conundrums and Predicaments in Psychotherapy and Psychoanalysis: The Clinical Moments Project*, ed. R. Tuch and L. Kuttnauer, London: Routledge, 222–41.

Harris, A. (2011), "The Relational Tradition: Landscape and Canon," *Journal of the American Psychoanalytic Association*, 59: 701–36.

Hartmann, H. (1950), "Comments on the Psychoanalytic Theory of the Ego," *Psychoanalytic Study of the Child* 5: 74–96.

Hartmann, H. (1965), *Essays on Ego Psychology*, New York: International Universities Press.

Hartmann, H., Kris, E., and Loewenstein, R. (1946), "Comments on the Formation of Psychic Structure," in *Psychoanalytic Study of the Child 24*, ed. R. S. Eissler et al., London: Hogarth, 11–38.

Heidegger, M. (1927), *Being and Time*, trans. J. Macquarrie and E. Robinson, New York: Harper Perennial.

Heimann, P. (1950), "On Countertransference," *International Journal of Psychoanalysis*, 31: 81–4.

Hertz, N. (1979), "Freud and the Sandman," in *Textual Strategies: Perspectives in Post-Structuralist Criticism*, ed. J. V. Harari, Ithaca, NY: Cornell University Press, 296–321.

Hinze, E. (2015), "What Do We Learn in Psychoanalytic Training?" *International Journal of Psychoanalysis*, 96: 755–71.

Hirsch, I. (2008), *Coasting in the Countertransference: Conflicts of Self-Interest between Analyst and Patient*, London: Routledge.

Hoffman, I. Z. (1983), "The Patient as Interpreter of the Analyst's Experience," *Contemporary Psychoanalysis*, 19: 389–422.

Hoffman, I. Z. (1994), "Dialectical Thinking and Therapeutic Action in the Psychoanalytic Process," *Psychoanalytic Quarterly*, 63: 187–218.

Hoffman, I. Z. (1996), "The Intimate and Ironic Authority of the Psychoanalyst's Presence," *Psychoanalytic Quarterly*, 65: 102–136.

Jacobs, T. J. (1986), "On Countertransference Enactments," *Journal of the American Psychoanalytic Association*, 34: 289–308.

Jacobs, T. J. (1991), *The Use of the Self: Countertransference and Communication in the Analytic Setting*, New York: International University Press.

Jaffe, J. and Feldstein, S. (1970), *Rhythms of Dialogue*, New York: Academic Press.

Joseph, B. (1971), "A Clinical Contribution to the Analysis of Perversion," *International Journal of Psychoanalysis*, 52: 441–9.

Joseph, B. (1985), "Transference: The Total Situation," *International Journal Psychoanalysis*, 66: 447–54.

Joseph, B. (1989), *Psychic Equilibrium and Psychic Change: Selected Papers of Betty Joseph*, ed. M. Feldman and E. B. Spillius, London: Routledge.

Kahneman, D. (2011), *Thinking Fast and Slow*, New York: Farrar, Straus and Giroux.

Kattlove, S. (2016), "Acknowledging the 'Analyst as Person:' A Developmental Achievement," *Journal of the American Psychoanalytic Association*, 64: 1207–16.

Kennedy, R. (2000), "Becoming a Subject: Some Theoretical and Clinical Issues," *International Journal of Psychoanalysis*, 81: 875–92.

Kirshner, L. (2005), "Rethinking Desire: The Objet Petit a in Lacanian Theory," *Journal of the American Psychoanalytic Association*, 53: 83–102.

Kirshner, L. (2011), "Neutrality and the Ethics of Desire," Paper presented at the meeting of the American Psychoanalytic Association, January 13, New York.

Kirshner, L. (2012), "Toward an Ethics of Psychoanalysis: A Critical Reading of Lacan's *Ethics*," *Journal of the American Psychoanalytic Association*, 60: 1223–42.

Kite, J. (2008), "Ideas of Influence: The Impact of the Analyst's Character on the Analysis," *Psychoanalytic Quarterly*, 77: 1075–104.

Kite, J. (2016), "The Fundamental Ethical Ambiguity of the Analyst-As-Person," *Journal of the American Psychoanalytic Association*, 64: 1153–71.

Kohut, H. (1971), *The Analysis of the Self: A Systematic Approach to the Treatment of Naricisstic Personality Disorders*. New York: International Universities Press.

Kojeve, A. ([1947] 1980), *Introduction to the Reading of Hegel*, trans. J. H. Nichols, Ithaca, NY: Cornell University Press.
Kravis, N. (2017), "The Googled and Googling Analyst," *Journal of the American Psychoanalytic Association*, 65: 799–818.
Kristeva, J. ([2007] 2010), "Speech in Psychoanalysis: From Symbols to the Flesh and Back," in *Reading French Psychoanalysis*, ed. D. Birksted-Breen, S. Flanders, and A. Gibeault, London: Routledge, 421–34.
Kristeva, J. (2014), "Reliance, or Maternal Eroticism," *Journal of the American Psychoanalytic Association*, 62: 69–86.
Lacan, J. ([1948] 2002), "Aggressiveness in Psychoanalysis," in *Écrits: The First Complete Edition in English*, trans. B. Fink, New York: Norton, 88–101.
Lacan, J. ([1949] 2002), "The Mirror Stage and the Formation of the *I* Function as Revealed in Psychoanalytic Experience," in *Écrits: The First Complete Edition in English*, trans. B. Fink, New York: Norton, 75–81.
Lacan, J. ([1953] 2002), "The Function and Field of Speech and Language in Psychoanalysis," in *Écrits: The First Complete Edition in English*, trans. B. Fink, New York: Norton, 197–268.
Lacan, J. ([1954] 2002), "Response to Jean Hyppolite's Commentary on Freud's 'Verneinung,'" in *Écrits: The First Complete Edition in English*, trans. B. Fink, New York: Norton, 197–268.
Lacan, J. ([1955–6] 1993), *The Seminar of Jacques Lacan: Book III. The Psychoses, 1955–1956*, ed. J.-A. Miller, trans. D. Porter, New York: Norton.
Lacan, J. ([1957–8] 2017), *The Seminar of Jacques Lacan: Book V. Formations of the Unconscious*, ed. J.-A. Miller, trans. R. Grigg, Cambridge: Polity Press.
Lacan, J. ([1959–60] 1992), *The Seminar of Jacques Lacan, Book VII. The Ethics of Psychoanalysis, 1959–1960*, ed. J.-A. Miller, trans. D. Porter, New York: Norton.
Lacan, J. ([1962–3] 2014), *The Seminar of Jacques Lacan, Book X. Anxiety*, ed. J.-A. Miller, trans. A. R. Price, Cambridge: Polity Press.
Lacan, J. ([1964] 1981), *The Four Fundamental Concepts of Psychoanalysis*, ed. J.-A. Miller, trans. A. Sherdan, New York: Norton.
Lagaay, A. (2008), "Between Sound and Silence: Voice in the History of Psychoanalysis," *E-pisteme*, 1: 53–62.
Laplanche, J. (1987), *New Foundations for Psychoanalysis*, trans. D. Macey, Cambridge, MA: Blackwell.
Laplanche, J. (1999), *Essays on Otherness*, London: Routledge.
Lear, J. (2003), "The Idea of a Moral Psychology: The Impact of Psychoanalysis on Philosophy in Britain," *International Journal of Psychoanalysis*, 84: 1351–61.
Lear, J. (2009), "Technique and Final Cause in Psychoanalysis: Four Ways of Looking at One Moment," *International Journal of Psychoanalysis*, 90: 1299–317.
Lear, J. (2011), *A Plea for Irony*, Cambridge, MA: Harvard University Press.

Lear, J. (2012), "Archimedean Desire: Commentary on Kirshner," *Journal of the American Psychoanalytic Association*, 60: 1243–9.

Leclaire, S. (1998), "On the Ear with Which One Ought to Listen," in *Psychoanalysing: On the Order of the Unconscious and the Practice of the Letter*, trans. P. Kamuf, Stanford, CA: Stanford University Press, 1–16.

Leikert, S. (2017), "'For Beauty Is Nothing but the Barely Endurable Onset of Terror': Outline of a General Psychoanalytic Aesthetics," *International Journal of Psychoanalysis*, 98: 657–81.

Levenson, E. ([1972] 1995), *Fallacy of Understanding*, Lanham, MD: Jason Aronson.

Levenson, E. ([1991] 2016), *The Purloined Self*, London: Routledge.

Lewis, M. (2016), *The Undoing Project: A Friendship That Changed Our Minds*, New York: Norton.

Lipton, S. (1977), "The Advantages of Freud's Technique as Shown in the Analysis of the Ratman," *International Journal of Psychoanalysis*, 58: 255–73.

Litowitz, B. (1999), "An Expanded Developmental Line for Negation: Rejection, Refusal, Denial," *Journal of the American Psychoanalytic Association*, 46: 121–48.

Litowitz, B. (2014), "From Switch-Words to Stitch-Words," *International Journal of Psychoanalysis*, 95: 3–14.

Loewald, H. (1980), *Papers on Psychoanalysis*, New Haven, CT: Yale University Press.

Markman, H. (2015), "A Pragmatic Approach to Bion's Late Work," *Journal of the American Psychoanalytic Association*, 63: 947–58.

McGuire, W., ed. (1974), Letter from Sigmund Freud to C. G. Jung, June 7, 1909, in *The Freud/Jung Letters: The Correspondence Between Sigmund Freud and C. G. Jung*. Princeton, NJ: Princeton University Press.

McLaughlin, J. T. (1991), "Clinical and Theoretical Aspects of Enactment," *Journal of the American Psychoanalytic Association*, 39: 595–614.

McWilliams, N. (2004), *Psychoanalytic Psychotherapy: A Practitioner's Guide*, New York: Guilford Press.

Mead, G. H. (1934), *Mind, Self, and Society: From the Standpoint of a Social-Behaviorist*, ed. C. W. Morris, Chicago, IL: University of Chicago Press.

Miller, D. A. (1981), *Narrative and Its Discontents: Problems of Closure in the Traditional Novel*, Princeton, NJ: Princeton University Press.

Miller, D. A. (1988), *The Novel and the Police*, Berkeley: University of California Press.

Miller, D. A. (2013), "Hitchcock's Understyle: A Too-Close View of 'Rope,'" *Representations* 121: 1–30.

Money-Kyrle, R. E. (1956), "Normal Countertransference and Some of Its Deviations," *International Journal Psychoanalysis*, 37: 360–6.

Morris, H. (2016), "The Analyst's Offer," *Journal of the American Psychoanalytic Association*, 64: 1173–87.

Moss, D. (2016), "The Insane Look of the Bewildered, Half-Broken Animal," *Journal of the American Psychoanalytic Association*, 64: 345–60.
Muller, F. (2016), "The Dialogical Self in Psychoanalysis," *Psychoanalytic Quarterly*, 85: 929–61.
Mulligan, D. (2017), "The Storied Analyst: Desire and Persuasion in the Clinical Vignette," *Psychoanalytic Quarterly*, 86: 811–33.
Nancy, J. and Lacoue-Labarthe, Philippe (1992), *The Title of the Letter: A Reading of Lacan*, Albany: SUNY Press.
Nobus, D. (2016), "For a New Gaya Scienza of Psychoanalysis," Division/Review, 15:17–23.
Ogden, T. H. (1994), "The Analytic Third: Working Intersubjectively with Clinical Facts," *International Journal of Psychoanalysis*, 75: 3–19.
Ogden, T. H. (1997), *Reverie and Interpretation: Sensing Something Human*, New York: Jason Aronson.
Ogden, T. H. (2000), "The Dialectically Constituted/Decentered Subject of Psychoanalysis," in *Psychoanalysis at Its Limits: Navigating the Post-Modern Turn*, ed. C. Spezzano and A. Elliott, London: Free Association Books, 203–38.
Ogden, T. H. (2015), "On Bion's 'Notes on Memory and Desire,'" *Psychoanalytic Quarterly*, 84: 285–306.
Ogden, T. H. (2016), "On Language and Truth in Psychoanalysis," *Psychoanalytic Quarterly*, 04. 411–26.
Ogden, T. H. and Gabbard, G. (2010), "The Lure of the Symptom in Psychoanalytic Treatment," *Journal of the American Psychoanalytic Association*, 58: 533–44.
Oldoini, M. G. (2019), "Abusive Relations and Traumatic Development: Marginal Notes on a Clinical Case," *Psychoanalytic Quarterly*, 88(2): 251–75.
Opatow, B. (1997), "The Real Unconscious: Psychoanalysis as a Theory of Consciousness," *Journal of the American Psychoanalytic Association*, 45: 865–90.
Parsons, M. (2014), *Living Psychoanalysis: From Theory to Experience*, East Sussex: Routledge.
Peters, J. D. (1999), *Speaking into the Air: A History of the Idea of Communication*, Chicago, IL: University of Chicago Press.
Pizer, S. (1992), "The Negotiation of Paradox in the Analytic Process," *Psychoanalytic Dialogues*, 2: 215–40.
Poland, W. (1992), "Transference: 'An Original Creation,'" *Psychoanalytic Quarterly*, 61: 185–205.
Pontalis, J.-B. (1981), *Frontiers in Psychoanalysis: Between the Dream and Psychic Pain*, trans. C. P. Cullen, New York: International Universities Press.
Purcell, S. D. (2004), "The Analyst's Theory: A Third Source of Counter-Transference," *International Journal of Psychoanalysis*, 85: 635–52.
Purcell, S. D. (2014), "Becoming Related: The Education of a Psychoanalyst," *Psychoanalytic Quarterly*, 83: 783–802.

Rabin, M. (1998), "Psychology and Economics," *Journal of Economic Literature*, 36: 11–46.
Racker, H. (1957), "The Meanings and Use of Counter-Transference," *Psychoanalytic Quarterly*, 26: 303–57.
Racker, H. (1968), *Transference and Countertransference*, New York: International University Press.
Rader, R. (1974), "Fact, Theory, and Literary Explanation," *Critical Inquiry*, 1(2): 245–72.
Reed, G. S. (2002), Review of *The Work of the Negative*, *Journal of the American Psychoanalytic Association*, 50: 343–8.
Reis, B. (2010), "Enactive Fields: An Approach to Interaction in the Kleinian-Bionian Model: Commentary on Paper by Lawrence J. Brown," *Psychoanalytic Dialogues*, 20: 695–703.
Renik, O. (1992), "Use of the Analyst as a Fetish," *Psychoanalytic Quarterly*, 61: 542–63.
Renik, O. (1993a), "Analytic Interaction: Conceptualizing Technique in Light of the Analyst's Irreducible Subjectivity," *Psychoanalytic Quarterly*, 62: 553–71.
Renik, O. (1993b), "Countertransference Enactment and the Psychoanalytic Process," in *Psychic Structure and Psychic Change: Essays in Honor of Robert Wallerstein, M.D.*, ed. M. J. Horowitz, O. F. Kernberg, and E. M. Weinshel, Madison, CT: International Universities Press, 135–58.
Renik, O. (2000), "Subjectivity and Unconsciousness," *Journal of Analytical Psychology*, 45: 3–20.
Renik, O. (2003), "Standards and Standardization," *Journal of the American Psychoanalytic Association*, 51: 43–55.
Renik, O. (2006), *Practical Psychoanalysis: A Guide for Clinicians*, New York: Other Press.
Ricouer, (1977), "The Question of Proof in Freud's Psychoanalytic Writings," *Journal of the American Psychoanalytic Association*, 25: 835–71.
Rieff, P. (1959), *Freud: Mind of the Moralist*, Chicago, IL: University of Chicago Press.
Rieff, P. (1966), *The Triumph of the Therapeutic: The Uses of Faith after Freud*, Chicago, IL: University of Chicago Press.
Rothstein, A. (1999), "Some Implications of the Analyst Feeling Disturbed When Working with Disturbed Patients," *Psychoanalytic Quarterly*, 68: 541–58.
Roudinesco, E. (2003), "The Mirror Stage: An Obliterated Archive," in *The Cambridge Companion to Lacan*, ed. J.-M. Rabaté, Cambridge: Cambridge University Press, 25–34.
Roussillon, R. (2011), *Primitive Agony and Symbolization*, London: Karnac.
Ruti, M. (2012), *The Singularity of Being: Lacan and the Immortal Within*, New York: Fordham University Press.
Schafer, R. (1976), *A New Language for Psychoanalysis*, New Haven, CT: Yale University Press.

Schafer, R. (1983), *The Analytic Attitude*, New York: Basic Books.
Schafer, R., ed. (1997), *The Contemporary Kleinians of London*, Madison, CT: International Universities Press.
Schafer, R. (2007), *Tragic Knots in Psychoanalysis*, London: Karnac.
Schafer, R. (2009), "The Countertransference of Feeling Frustrated," in *Tragic Knots in Psychoanalysis: New Papers on Psychoanalysis*, London: Karnac, 71–84.
Schlesinger, H. J. (1995), "The Process of Interpretation and the Moment of Change," *Journal of the American Psychoanalytic Association*, 43: 663–8.
Searle, J. R. (1983), *Intentionality: An Essay in the Philosophy of Mind*, Cambridge: Cambridge University Press.
Searle, J. R. (2001), *Rationality in Action*, Cambridge: MIT Press.
Seligman, S. (2018), "Illusion as a Basic Psychic Principle: Winnicott, Freud, Oedipus, and Trump," *Journal of the American Psychoanalytic Association*, 66: 263–88.
Sharpe, E. F. (1950), *Collected Papers on Psychoanalysis*, London: Hogarth Press.
Shulman, M. (2016), "The Analyst's Pleasures," *Journal of the American Psychoanalytic Association*, 64: 697–727.
Smith, J. H. (1991), *Arguing with Lacan: Ego Psychology and Language*, New Haven, CT: Yale University Press.
Sorosky, A. D., Baran, A., and Pannor, R. (1979), *The Adoption Triangle: Sealed or Open Records and How They Affect Adoptees, Birth Parents, and Adoptive Parents*, Ann Arbor, MI: Anchor Press.
Spillius, E. (1988), *Melanie Klein Today: Developments in Theory and Practice, Vol. 2: Mainly Practice*, London: Routledge.
Spillius, E. (1992), "Clinical Experiences of Projective Identification," in *Clinical Lectures on Klein and Bion*, ed. R. Anderson, London: Tavistock/Routledge, 59–73.
Spillius, E. (2007), *Encounters with Melanie Klein: Selected Papers of Elizabeth Spillius*, London: Routledge.
Spillius, E. and O'Shaughnessy, E. (2012), *Projective Identification: The Fate of a Concept*, London: Routledge.
Steiner, J. (1993), *Psychic Retreats: Pathological Organizations in Psychotic, Neurotic, and Borderline Patients*, London: Routledge.
Steiner, J. (2011), "The Numbing Feeling of Reality," *Psychoanalytic Quarterly*, 80: 73–90.
Stern, D. B. (2018), *The Infinity of the Unsaid: Unformulated Experience, Language, and the Non-Verbal*, Oxford: Routledge.
Sterne, L. ([1767] 1940), *The Life and Opinions of Tristram Shandy, Gentleman*, ed. J. Work, Indianapolis, IN: Bobbs-Merrill.
Stevens, W. (1954), "The Snowman," in *The Collected Poems of Wallace Stevens*, New York: Knoft, 9.
Swift, J. ([1704] 2010), *A Tale of a Tub and Other Works*, ed. Marcus Walsh, Cambridge: Cambridge University Press.

Tower, L. (1956), "Countertransference," *Journal of the American Psychoanalytic Association*, 4: 224–55.
Tversky, A. and Kahneman, D. (1974), "Judgement under Uncertainty: Heuristics and Biases," *Science*, New Series, 185: 1124–31.
Waelder, R. (1936), "The Principle of Multiple Function: Observations on Over-Determination," *Psychoanalytic Quarterly*, 5: 45–62.
Webb, R. E. and Sells, M. A. (1995), "Lacan and Bion: Psychoanalysis and the Mystical Language of 'Unsaying,'" *Theory Psychology*, 5: 195–215.
Webster, J. (2011), *The Life and Death of Psychoanalysis*, London: Karnac Books.
Weiss, J. (1993), *How Psychotherapy Works: Process and Technique*, New York: Guilford Press.
Weiss, J., Sampson, H., and The Mount Zion Psychotherapy Research Group (1986), *The Psychoanalytic Process: Theory, Clinical Observations and Empirical Research*, New York: Guilford Press.
Williams, B. (1985), *Ethics and the Limits of Philosophy*, London: Fontana.
Wilson, M. (1986), "'And Let Me Go On': Tristram Shandy, Lacanian Theory, and the Dialectic of Desire," *Psychoanalytic Contemporary Thought*, 9(3): 335–72.
Wilson, M. (2003), "The Analyst's Desire and the Problem of Narcissistic Resistances," *Journal of the American Psychoanalytic Association*, 51: 397–421.
Wilson, M. (2006), "'Nothing Could Be Further from the Truth': The Role of Lack in the Analytic Process," *Journal of the American Psychoanalytic Association*, 54: 397–421.
Wilson, M. (2010), "Putting Practice into Theory: Making the Training Analyst System Coherent," *Journal of the American Psychoanalytic Association*, 58: 287–311.
Wilson, M. (2012), "The Flourishing Analyst, Responsibility, and Psychoanalytic Ethics: Commentary on Kirshner," *Journal of the American Psychoanalytic Association*, 60: 1251–8.
Wilson, M. (2013), "Desire and Responsibility: The Ethics of Countertransference Experience," *Psychoanalytic Quarterly*, 82: 435–76.
Wilson, M. (2016), "The Desire for Therapeutic Gain: Commentary on Chused's 'An Analyst's Uncertainty and Fear,'" *Psychoanalytic Quarterly*, 85: 857–65.
Wilson, M. (2018), "The Analyst as Listening-Accompanist: Desire in Bion and Lacan," *Psychoanalytic Quarterly*, 87: 237–64.
Winnicott, D. W. (1956), "On Transference," *International Journal of Psychoanalysis*, 37: 386–88.
Winnicott, D. W. (1969), "The Use of an Object," *International Journal of Psychoanalysis*, 50: 711–16.
Wollheim, R. (1993), Personal communication.
Woolf, V. ([1927] 2019), *To the Lighthouse*, London: Penguin Classics.
Žižek, S. (2007), "Lacan: At What Point Is He Hegelian?" trans. R. Butler and S. Stevens, retrieved from http://www.lacan.com/zizlacan1.htm (July 10, 2011).

# Index

Abrams, S. 49, 52
absence xiii, xiv, 24, 56, 59, 86, 88, 96, 101, 176
   and presence 84, 88
action (analyst's) 52, 97, 102, 174, 182–4
   analyst's responsibility for 148
   as an object of judgment 158–62
   as a carrier of judgment 158, 159, 162–5
   enactment xii–xiii, 18, 54, 120, 122, 166–8
   ethics of 99, 115 n.24, 119–21, 145, 146
   The Ethical Foundation of Analytic Action 155–69
   fading as subject, unthought, absence xiii, 166–8
   Lacan on 119, 147, 155
   Renik on 185
   Schafer's concept of 76, 155, 184
*Adoption Triangle, The* (Sorosky) 8
affect intolerance xxi
Aguayo, J. 102 n.6, 115 n.23
Akerlof, G. 41 n.12
*All in the Family* 5
alpha function 105
Altieri, C.
   articulation and subjective emergence 3, 10
   example 174
   exemplary/exemplification 174, 176, 177
   on Hamlet 174–5
   values 174
American Ego Psychology 10, 50, 51, 54, 55, 58, 67, 173
   speaking as "street talk" 13
   *see also* one-person psychology

American Psychoanalytic Association 32, 49, 56, 166
"Analysis Terminable and Interminable" 200
analyst(s)
   as fetish 200–2
   as innkeeper 15–30
   judgment 101, 159–61
   lacking position 76–81
   as listening-accompanist 112–14
   proleptic transformation 172, 177, 190, 192, 194
   resistance 61–6
   "The Analyst's Desire and the Problem of Narcissistic Resistances" 56
analyst's position
   anticipatory xvi, 80, 125, 165, 168, 172, 199
   at-one-ment xvi, 99, 109
   basic working conditions 80, 131, 167, 168
   caretaking 16, 17, 27, 96, 112
   curator of space xvi, xviii, xxii, 47, 80, 94
   as dislocated 47, 165
   futural xvi, xviii, 54, 97, 102, 125, 147, 165, 168, 171–83, 189, 199, 207, 208
   gyroscopic xvi, xviii, 81, 88, 97, 125, 147, 173, 199, 207, 209
   as (falsely) heroic xxi, 116, 201, 209
   as innkeeper xvi, 15–17, 95, 195, 207, 209
   lacking xviii, xxii, 38 n.9, 57, 75–81, 94, 108, 115 n.25, 116, 173, 209
   and listening 94, 165
   as listening-accompanist 95–117

as positive presence 80, 84, 87, 88
analytic attitude 78, 93–4
analytic conviction 32
analytic desire 1, 27, 28, 30, 32, 51, 63, 70, 72, 94, 108–10, 114, 116, 130, 133, 173, 199
analytic field/field theory, and paranoia 125, 134
analytic identity 32
analytic relationship xii, 3, 20 n.5, 25, 27, 28, 30, 52, 63, 126, 146, 156, 158 n.5, 164, 179, 189, 200–2, 204–8
    and illusion 200, 201, 202, 203
    reality of 83, 109, 110, 201
    as *sui generis* 206, 208
analytic third 146
anchoring 40–1
anthropomorphic language 183
anthropomorphism 183
anticipation *vs.* prediction 194
Applegarth, A. xxvi, 12
*Après-coup* 55, 97, 157, 172 n.2, 185, 193
Aristotle 58, 121, 158 n.6
Arlow, J. xxii, 12, 181
Armstrong, L. 113
articulation and subjective emergence 3, 10, 22
at-one-ment xvi, 99, 109
"Attacks on Linking" 104
*Attention and Interpretation* 82
Austin, J.L.
    "perlocutionary force" 23
availability of instances 39–40

bad faith xii
    and *ressentiment* xii, xiii, 135n8
Balliett, W. 113
Barthes, R. 10, 25
Baxter, C.
    all the "talking forks" 196
    "the logic of unveiling" 43 n.13, 46 n.16, 176
Beebe, B. 113 n.21

Benjamin, J.
    "doer-done to" 64, 78, 138
    and moral third 125, 146 n.12
    and surrender 66
    *Beyond the Pleasure Principle* 107 n.14, 182
Bion, W.
    alpha-function 105
    at-one-ment xvi, 99, 109
    "Attacks on Linking" 104
    *Attention and Interpretation* 82
    caesura 104, 112
    confusion of desire and wish 116
    on desire 99–102
    on emotional experience 98–100, 103, 105, 107, 109, 112
    on language 98–9, 103–6, 109, 112
    "language of achievement" 104, 104 n.8
    Los Angeles seminars 100, 103, 105
    on memory and desire 38 n.9, 99–101, 116
    negative capability 99, 104
    "O" 98–100, 105, 115
    "transformations in 'O' " 115
Bloom, H. 124, 124 n.3
Bott-Spillius, E. 55
boundary violations 167 n.8
British Independent Group 77
Britton, R. 55, 116
Browning, R.
    "My Last Duchess" 9
Busch, F. 87
Butler, J. xxv, 2, 3

caesura 104, 112
Carmichael, H.
    "Stardust" 83
Carson, A. 95
Cartesian subject 58
Casement, P.
    *Learning from our Mistakes* 78
    *Learning from the Patient* 78
Casterline, F. "Cas" 6

# Index

Caston, J.
"the bond of safe company" 17, 20, 23, 25, 26, 28, 29
Catlett, "Big" Sid 113
causality 183
Chetrit-Vatine, V.
  asymmetry of analytic relationship 20 n.5, 158 n.5
  ethical responsibility for the other xvii, 96, 158 n.5, 164
  *The Ethical Seduction of the Analytic Situation* xvii, 18
  matricial space xvii, 18, 20
  power of the face/interpellation 18
  and transference 20
Civitarese, G. 163, 164, 174 n.3
clinical cases
  Byron 123 n.2, 148–53
  Evan 75, 76, 81, 89–93
  Genevieve 26, 27
  Joan 25–30, 44 n.14, 93
  Luna 186–90, 193, 194
  Molly 177–80, 189, 190
  Paul 23–7
  Robert 66–73
  Thomas 190–3
clinical impasse xi, xiii, 43, 65, 71, 73, 139
  trauma 56
  unpleasure and xii, 139
clinical writing 43, 175
  analyst as hero 44–5
  vignette as short-story 45
closural nature of narrative 42–6
cognitive bias xv, 37–41
  anchoring
    nature of happiness 40
    reference level 40
  availability of instances
    false correlation 39
    near-term bias 39
  first impressions 39
  "Judgment Under Uncertainty: Heuristics and Biases" 38

Kahneman, D. xv, 33, 37–41
  "pattern recognition" 38
  prior probability 38
  representativeness 38, 39, 41, 42
  Tversky, A. xv, 33, 37–41
colonization xiii, 53–6
  of patient's mind 69
  of patient's text 63
conditions of satisfaction 133–49, 154, 163
  judgment of action and 161–2
  narrative and xv, 31
confusion of self and other 62, 134, 138, 144, 152
consultation 41–2
containing 20, 87, 98, 127, 202
contingency, accident 119, 178–9, 194
patient's singularity xxii, 17
conversion to psychoanalysis 32
Cooper, S.
  and analyst's narcissism 131
  and externalizing responsibility 139
  and "new bad object" 79
Corporal Trim's "flourish with his stick" 21, *21*, 199
Cossette, J. 4, 5, 8, 13, 14
countertransference xii, 122
  as activity 151
  analyst's ethical responsibility for 20, 103
  and desire xii, xix, xxi, 13, 57 n.3, 102, 116, 119–54, 162
  dual relation 125, 137, 139–44, 151
  enactment 54, 120, 122, 166–8
  logic of experience 131–4
  narrow view 128–9
  and projective identification 125–7
  Racker, H. on 116, 124, 128, 134, 136, 139, 140
  and resentment xii, 65
  talion law 125, 134, 137, 139–44, 151
  wider view 125–8

desire
  analyst's xvii
    as "force-element" 98, 103
    futural position 97, 172
    ideal position xix, 98, 100, 108, 109
    signifier-moments and 111
  and contemporary psychoanalytic landscape xix–xxii
  countertransference (*see* countertransference)
  dissatisfaction and xii, 52, 119, 134, 136, 137, 141, 151
  distinguished from wish xiii, 56, 97–8
  and ending of analysis 195–210
  forever nature of 199
  and Fort! Da! xiv, 56, 83, 176, 178, 179
  imaginary and xiii, xvii, xxi, 22, 31, 37, 41, 42, 56, 101, 116, 117, 137, 148, 152, 199
  "indestructible" nature 97, 198
  Lacan on 102–3
  lack and xiv, xviii, 47, 56, 57, 59, 61, 75–94, 98, 111 n.18, 123, 146, 147, 207
  and psychoanalytic training/education xxiv
  for recognition 61, 62, 64, 65, 73, 84, 131, 146, 152, 165, 174
  reduced to wish 33, 97, 117
  responsibility, and analytic action 144–8
  satisfaction and xi, xv, 3, 31, 37, 59, 72, 82, 101, 116, 133, 135, 138, 141, 143, 149, 154, 161, 162, 163, 182
  and space xvi, xviii, xx, xxii, 11, 27, 47, 64, 65, 72, 73, 78–80, 84, 86–8, 94–6, 112, 134, 158, 173, 177, 180, 184, 185, 193, 197, 206–8
  tragic dimension 185
  wanting xii, xiv, 10, 25, 50, 84, 92, 102, 124, 130, 135, 137, 140, 151–3, 166, 173
  and wish 56–8
dialectic/dialectical 35, 54, 55, 78 n.2, 82, 84, 146 n.12, 153, 165, 168, 172 n.2, 203, 208
dispositions 207
"Dream of Irma's Injection" 81
"Dream of the Botanical Monograph" 108
dual relation
  contested analytic field 66
  imaginary relation and 137
  inherently reversible/reversibility of 62
  and judgement under uncertainty (bias) 42
  paranoid analytic field 125
  and resistance xiii, 61–6, 73, 88, 137–9, 148–51, 188
  talion law and 125, 128 n.5, 137–44, 138 n.9, 148, 152
  undecidability and 88
Dunn, J. xxiv, 89
Dylan, B. 171

ego
  and the "ego's audits" 36, 37, 60
  gestalt totality 36
  imaginary structure 41
  and narcissism 31–48
  specular nature 36
  "squaring of ego's audits" 36, 60
  as unstable narcissistic structure 36
*Ego and the Id, The* 34
Eidetic reduction 100, 100 n.4
Elise, D. xvi, xxiv
ending of analysis (termination) 195–210
ends of analysis 159–61, 169, 205
eros xiv, 56
ethical unconscious 114–17

ethics
and analytic action xiii, 99, 115, 115 n.24, 155–69
Antigone 145
Chetrit-Vatine, V. xvii
and countertransference 119–54
and end of analysis 199
and "fading of the subject" 166–8
Lacan, J. on xvii, 52, 99, 153
Lear, J. 99 n.3
matricial space and 26–30
morality, difference from xiii, 157
Morris, H. 17 n.3, 167
responsibility
and desire xii, 119–54
and limits of self-knowledge 2
for the other xvii, 17, 19, 23, 30, 96, 158 n.5, 164
Schafer, R. 155, 158 n.4
Evans, D. 85, 106 n.12
exemplary moment 171–94
Altieri, C. and 174, 176, 177
and the futural xvi, 171, 174–7

fading of the subject 166–8
Faimberg, H. 94
on countertransference position and unpleasure 132
"listening to listening" 54, 78, 78 n.2
Feldman, M. 55, 124, 128, 128 n.5, 132, 132 n.6, 136
case of Mr. G. 140–43
Ferenczi, S.
on "proper ending of an analysis" 200, 209
and thought transference xx
Ferro, A. 55, 122
*Field of Dreams* 13
figurative language 130, 182, 183, 185, 202
Fineman, J. xxiv, 11
Fink, B. 147 n.13
Fish, S., on belief 64 n.7
Fonagy, P. 83

Fort! Da! xiv, 56, 83, 176, 178, 179
and desire xiv, 56, 83, 176, 178, 179
and space 84
and the structure of the subject xiv, 83, 178
Foucault, M.
"What is an Author?" 10
*Four Fundamental Concepts of Psychoanalysis, The* 102
freedom of speech 3
Freud, S.
"Analysis Terminable and Interminable" 200
*Beyond the Pleasure Principle* 107 n.14, 182
"Dream of Irma's Injection" 81
"Dream of the Botanical Monograph" 108
*The Ego and the Id* 34
Fort! Da! xiv, 56, 83, 176, 178, 179
*The Interpretation of Dreams* 4, 81
*Joke Book* 4
navel of dream and lack 81, 82, 168
*Nebenmensch* 28
"On Narcissism" 34, 58
*Wunsch* 49, 97
Freud and Breuer
*Studies in Hysteria* 43
Friedman, L. 49, 51–3, 72–3, 115 n.24, 155
on nature of analytic love 204

Gabbard, G. 64–8, 208
and the ungrateful patient 60
Gillespie, D. 113
Glover, E. xviii
Goldberg, A.
on misunderstanding 78
Goldberg, P. xxv, 20
*Grateful Dead*
Dark Star xvii
Graves, R. 1
Gray, P.
and American ego psychology 50

"close process monitoring" 50, 51
resistance analysis 72
Green, A.
  analytic object 144
  on Bion 82, 86
  *The Work of the Negative* 83, 85, 86
Greenberg, J. 98 n.2, 145
  on "guiding fictions" 163–4
  and the nature of belief 164
Greenson, R. 18 n.4, 19, 20
Grossman, L. xxiv, 76, 77, 166
Grossman and Simon
  on anthropomorphic language 183
  critique of ego-psychology 173
Grotstein, J. 104 n.8, 115, 115 n.23

Hamilton, A. 5
*Hamlet* 67, 174–5
Harms, D.
  case of Jake 45, 46
Hartmann, H.
  distinction between ego and self 58
  ego psychology 58, 183
Heidegger, M.
  *Dasein*, Being 56, 172
Hewitson, O. xxv, 107 n.14
Hirsch, I.
  on analyst's difficulty ending treatments 200
  *Coasting in the Countertransference* 41 n.10
Hoffman, I. 51, 54, 64
Houston, B. Dr. 103 n.7
Hunter, R. 14, 208

idealization 32, 33, 52, 187, 200 32, 33, 52, 187, 200
The Imaginary xiii, xv n.1, xvii, xxi, 22, 31, 37, 41, 42, 56, 101, 110 n.17, 116, 117, 137, 148, 152, 199
Imaginary order 31
Imaginary register xiii, xv n.1, 41, 56, 116, 137

*International Journal of Psychoanalysis* 87, 174 n.3
*Interpretation of Dreams, The* 4, 81
intuition 98, 99, 105, 109, 110, 111, 116

Jaspers, K.
  *General Psychopathology* 37, 40
  "relation of understanding" 37, 39, 40
*Joke Book* 4
Joseph, B.
  "A Clinical Contribution to the Analysis of Perversion" 63
  bias toward positive presence 87
  and Busch, F. 87
  and dual-relation resistance 88
  and Gabbard, G.O. 64, 65
  and the master's discourse 54
  on transference as "total situation" 86
judgment under uncertainty 42
Jung, C.G.
  and Sabina Spielrein 121
  and thought transference xx

Kahneman, D. xv, 33, 37–40
*Thinking Fast and Slow* 37
Kennedy, R. 73, 106 n.12
Kirshner, L.
  analytic ethics 115 n.24
  on desire 115 n.24
Kite, J. 49, 52, 165
Klein, M. 24
  compared to Lacan 24, 81, 88
  on countertransference 125, 126, 131, 137, 153
  on object relation 81, 86, 88
Kleinian school/London Kleinians
  and the analyst's desire xiii, 63
  and clinical impasse xiii, 56
  colonization (of SFPI) xiii, 55
  countertransference xiii, 63, 124
  and dual relation resistance xiii, 88

and ego psychology 54, 55, 57, 86
misrecognition xiii, 89
Kohut, H. 53, 78
Kravis, N. 177, 205
Kris, E.
    "pattern recognition" 38
Kristeva, J.
    " 'Speech in psychoanalysis': From Symbols to Flesh and Back" 22, 23, 23 n.7

Lacan, J.
    absolute difference xviii, xix
    *agalma* xviii, 200, 201
    *Anxiety* (seminar X) 4 n.1, 200 n.4
    Big Other 21, 85, 145
    critique of xiii, 37, 38, 116–17, 121, 137, 146–8, 199
    desire of the analyst xvii, xviii, 96–8, 100–3
    discourse of mastery xviii
    *Ethics of Psychoanalysis* 119, 144, 155
    and Fort! Da! 83
    *The Four Fundamental Concepts of Psychoanalysis/Seminar 11* xvii, 102
    Imaginary order 31
    intuition, skepticism of 98–9, 110, 116
    "I shelter my responsibility" 107
    lack in the other xviii, 84, 85
    on language 85, 98, 99, 103, 106–9
    limitations of 106
    Maltese falcon xviii, 209
    on meeting Bion 102
    mirror stage xv, 30–47, 53, 66, 124, 173
    negative theology 89
    *objet petit a*, object cause(s) of desire 200
    on representation 83, 98, 107
    sea-captain passage 107, 108, 110

*sinthome* xvii, 208
speech relation/speaking subject xvii, 21, 28 n.11, 99, 106–12, 116
talking cure 4, 20
"The Function and Field of Speech and Language in Psychoanalysis" 110
and *Tristram Shandy* 198, 199
lack
    analyst's inhabiting the position of xxii, 38 n.9, 80, 88, 111 n.18
    and the analyst's mistakes 78, 79
    and basic working conditions 80, 81, 146
    and bias toward absence xiv
    and desire xiv, xviii, 56, 57, 59, 61, 75, 88, 98, 111 n.18, 147
    and navel of the dream 82, 168
    in the other xviii, 84, 85, 91
    symbolic remainder 82–5
Lacoue-Labarthe, P. 89
Lagaay, A. 4 n.1
"language of achievement" 104, 104 n.8
Laplanche, J.
    and enigma of the message 22, 33 n.1
    and enigma of the other's desire 107 n.13, 205
    hollowed-out transference 27
    narcissistic closure 30, 32, 33, 57, 117
    primary anthropological situation 19
    "The Unfinished Copernican Revolution" 34 n.2
Lear, J.
    analytic ethics 160
    goal of analysis 160
    irony and 153
Leclaire, S. 55, 136
Levinson, E.
    *The Fallacy of Understanding* 54

*The Purloined Self* 54
Levi-Strauss, C.
   *bricoleur* 10
Lewis, M.
   *The Undoing Project* 37 n.7
Lipton, S 15 n.1
listening
   for the "other" 7, 84
Litowitz, B. xxiv
   on negation as a developmental line 83
   "stitch words" 26, 42
Loewald, H. 173
   mind as "temporal in nature" 184
Lure of plenitude 81, 91, 144 n. 11
   and obsessional structure 84–7

Markman, H.
   on Bion 104, 105
matricial space 17–21
   ethics of care xvii, 26–30
   responsibility for the other xvii, 23, 30
McWilliams, N. 172
Mead, G.H. 36 n.5, 178
meaning 183
   as lacking 80
   and structure 84
   and the symbolic 10–11
Melville, H. 3
Miller, D.A. (David) xxiv, 11, 45 n.15
   "too-close reading" 51
Milton, J. 3
Mirror stage xv, 30, 31, 33–7, 53, 66, 124, 173
   as identification 35, 53
   Joseph, B. and 124
   "relation of understanding" 35
   as temporal dialectic 35
   "The Mirror Stage as Formative of the I Function" 35
Morris, H.
   foundational ethics 17 n.3
   illusion 202, 203

living the real 167, 203, 204
"The Analyst's Offer" 17 n.3
Moss, D. xxiv
"The Insane Look of the Bewildered, Half-Broken Animal" 41
motive 183
Mulligan, D.
   analyst as detective and epic hero 44
   "The Storied Analyst: Desire and Persuasion in the Clinical Vignette" 44

Nancy, J.-L. 89
narcissism 34, 58
   narcissistic closure 30–47, 117
   natural narcissism 33, 58, 60
   *see also* ego; Mirror Stage
narrative
   closural nature of 42–6
   and "connecting the dots" 46
   importance of disruption 28, 46
   narcissistic investment in case of Jake 45–6
   psychoanalysis as fundamentally different from 43
navel of dream and lack 81, 82, 168
*Nebenmensch* 28
negative capability 99, 104
Nietzsche, F. xv
Nobus, D.
   "position of the analyst" 109, 113
nothing
   and desire 85, 93, 148, 168
   and lack 76, 79
   and Searle, J.R. (the gap) 82
   traumatic effects of 90
"Nothing could be further from the truth" xvi, 75–94
now-and-the-next 26, 30, 33, 42, 43, 46, 80, 94, 96, 99, 161–3, 166, 171, 172, 175, 179, 180 n.8, 185, 193, 207

"O" 98–100, 105, 115
  transformations in 115
object relation
  Klein on 81, 86
  Lacan on 81, 137
  nature of 81, 88–9
Ogden, T.
  on Bion 101, 105, 109–10, 115
  on "direct discourse" 105
  on dreaming/waking dreaming 109, 115
  "The Dialectically Constituted/ Decentered Subject of Psychoanalysis" 79
Oldoini, M.G. 172 n.1
one-person psychology 13, 120
ontology
  basis of the subject 147
  gap xx
  lack xiv
Opatow, B.
  re-finding lost object 6
  "The Real Unconscious" 58–9, 82, 83
  on wish-fulfillment 59
Other/Big Other
  enigma and 85, 107 n.13
  and fantasy 85
  lack in xviii, 84, 85, 91
  obsessional bias and 85
  and radical alterity xxi, 85

patient-as-person 27
patient's "affect intolerance" xxi
Peters, J.D.
  *A History of the Idea of Communication* xix, 105
  idea of communication xix, 105
  *see also* Speech
poesis
  futural nature of 180
  and insight 44
Poland, W. 49, 51, 179 n.8
Pontalis, J.-B. 59

prior probability 38
projective identification 86, 109, 129
  and the dual relation xiii, 125–7, 140, 144, 152
Prolepsis, proleptic
  unconscious xvi, xxi, 81, 171–94, 199, 207
psychoanalysis 40
  speech relation in 21–6
psychoanalytic conviction 32
psychoanalytic identity 32
Purcell, S.
  attenuated countertransference 89
  on psychoanalysis as a treatment 160

Rabin, M. 39
Racker, H.
  complimentary identifications 125
  on countertransference 116, 120, 124, 125, 130, 131, 134, 137–9, 141
  on desire 120, 124, 125, 130, 131, 134–7, 139, 140, 142
  talion law 137, 138
Rader, R. 9–11, 10 n.3
"rational" judgment 39
The real
  living the real (Morris, H.) 167, 168, 203, 204
  "O" 98, 115
  trauma and xxii, 56
  unsymbolizable 98
Reed, Gail on Andre Green 85
Reis, B. 185 n.12
relational tradition
  asymmetry 20
  missing the patient 78
relation of understanding 39
Renik, O. xii–xiii, 12, 36, 49, 51, 53, 143 n.10, 146, 155, 173
  on the analyst as fetish 200–2, 206
  on the analyst's irreducible subjectivity 54

on analytic action xii, 54
on countertansference 54, 122
on enactment xii, 54
on the goals of analysis 159–61
on the unconscious 180
representativeness (bias) 38–9
resistance 50
   analyst's xiii, 38 n.9, 49–73, 162
   and the analyst's desire xiii, 49–73
   Benjamin, J. and misrecognition and surrendering 66
   and bias toward presence 88
   clinical problems with the analysis of 49, 62
   dual relation and xiii, 66, 73, 88, 137–9, 148–51, 188
   Freud, S. and 43, 49, 50
   Friedman, L. and 49
   Gray, P. 50–2
   narcissistic basis of 62
   and unconscious ego defenses 50
Resistance: A Reevaluation, panel 49
reverie 98, 104 n.8, 105, 109, 116, 127, 147
Ricoeur, P. 185
Rieff, P. 156 n.1
Rivers, J. 1
Robertson, R. xix
Rothstein, A. 69
Roudinesco, E. 35 n.4
Rousillion, R. 183 n.11
Rudnytsky, P. xxv, 23 n.7
Ruti, M. xxii n.6, 108, 145

San Francisco Psychoanalytic Institute 12, 54 n.1
   colonization of 53–6
   institutional history 53–6
Sawtelle Field 6, 8
Schafer, R.
   action language 158 n.4, 184
   on analytic action 76
   on frustration 153

*A New Language for Psychoanalysis* 155
   on reification of unconscious content 184
Searle, J.
   and desire 82, 83, 133, 135
   and the "gap" 82, 83
selected fact *vs.* overvalued idea 116
self-knowledge 2
Seligman, S.
   on illusion 202, 203
sense impressions 110
Sharpe, E. 60
Shulman, M. 101, 102, 156
signifier 83, 106
   of the lack in Other 84
   moments 111
Silverstein, Shel
   *Missing Piece Looking for the Big O* 84
Smith, J.H. 61
Sorosky, A. 8
   *The Adoption Triangle* 8
   advice 8
   death 13
speech
   analyst as interlocutor 20, 25
   analyst's denial of
   and fallacy of split between word and body 3 n.8
   as "felt difference" 22–4, 27, 42
   and the innkeeper 17, 195–7, 209–10
   levels of abstraction 24
   relation xvii, xx, 20–8, 28 n.11, 30, 31, 42, 43, 78, 99, 106–12, 116, 207
   repurposed 27, 30
   signifier as open potential 108
   signifier *vs.* signified 83, 106
   "stitch words" 42
   "The Function and Field of Speech and Language in Psychoanalysis" 110

Steiner, J. 55, 116, 127, 145
Stern, D.
 "infinity of the unsaid" xvi, 199
 unformulated experience xvi
Sterne, L.
 *Tristram Shandy* 105 n.10
Stevens, W. 75
"Storied Analyst, The: Desire and Persuasion in the Clinical Vignette" 44
stranger, strangerness
 and analyst as innkeeper 15–16
 disruptions in analytic process 28
 *Nebenmensch* 28
 street talk 13
subject
 decentered 34 n.2, 78, 79, 159
 ontology 147
 structure of 84
 subjective destitution xiv, 93
Sullivan, H.S. 20
Swift, J. 15, 23
symbolic
 remainder 98
 stain 82
 and structure 110
symbolic castration 83, 94

Target, M. 83
theory as defense against recognition of analyst's desire 62 102
Tov, B.-S. 5
Tower, Lucia
 "countertransference" 200 n.4
transference
 Betty Joseph on 54–5, 63, 86
 interpretation of 55, 189, 204
 Lacan on xviii, 89, 95, 103, 108, 109 n.15, 116, 200
 as lure xviii, 89
 as repetition 127
trauma xii–xv, xx, xxii, xxiii, 28, 49, 53, 56, 69, 76, 90, 104, 117, 134, 138, 148, 151, 152, 169, 172 n.1, 176, 179, 187, 191
Tversky, A. xv, 33, 37–41

UC Berkeley, English Department 9
UCSF 9, 11
unconscious
 ethics and 114–17
 as nonsubstantive 114
 "pre-ontological" 99, 114
 proleptic nature of xvi, xxi, 81, 171–94, 199, 207
 reification and xxi, 180–2, 184, 185
understanding, as ideal relation 38
unrepresented mental states 176 n.6

voice xvii, xviii, xx, xxii, 1–15, 79, 152, 171, 197, 204
 cause of desire 5
 indelibility 5

Wallon, H.
 "mirror test" 35 n.4
Webster, J. xiv, 156
Weiss, J.
 pathogenic beliefs xxii
 as supervisor 169
Williams, B.
 "morality system" 157
Williams, T.
 *The Science of Hitting* 6
Wilson, J. 5
Wilson, M.
 "'and let me go on': *Tristram Shandy*, Lacanian Theory, and the Dialectic of Desire" 198, 199
 baseball/hitting 6
 father 5, 7, 11
 first analysis 12
Winnicott, D.W.
 false self 36

on interpreting and the limits of
    understanding 78
"On Transference" 77
"The Use of the Object" 11
transitional objects 11
wish
    Bion and 82, 93, 101, 109, 116

direct object and 95, 116
as distinguished from desire xiii,
    56, 97–8
Woolf, V.
    "Time Passes" 195
*work of the negative* 86
*Wunsch* 49, 97

www.ingramcontent.com/pod-product-compliance
Lightning Source LLC
Chambersburg PA
CBHW070029010526
44117CB00011B/1757